9·23·77

Good Housekeeping
Guide to Medicines and Drugs

Judith K. Jones MD PhD

Good Housekeeping Books
New York, New York

ISBN 0–87851–021–4

Library of Congress Catalogue Number 77–072363

About the Author

Judith K. Jones practices internal medicine and clinical pharmacology in San Francisco. She is Chief of the Division of Clinical Pharmacology at Presbyterian Hospital, Pacific Medical Center, and Assistant Clinical Professor of Medicine at University of California in San Francisco. She is also Adjunct Professor of Physiology and Pharmacology at the University of the Pacific School of Pharmacy, and a consultant to the U.S. Food and Drug Administration.

Special Editorial Advisers   1984565

Joseph E. Snyder, M.D., is Director of Medical Affairs at the Columbia-Presbyterian Medical Center in New York.

Peter Rheinstein is Head of Division of Drug Advertising, Food and Drug Administration, Department of Health, Education and Welfare.

Acknowledgements

The author wishes to express her gratitude to Dr. Donald Shirachi, Dr. John Pech, Dr. Ed Elzarian, Dr. Kenneth Low, Ms Sharon Mauldin and Ms Martha Lowery for their help in researching and reviewing the information contained in this book.

Contents

Contents

Foreword

As a physician and pharmacologist with a long-time interest in educating other physicians, medical and pharmacy students, paramedical health workers (and my own patients) about how medicines act and work, the opportunity to prepare an everyday guide for the larger public was a welcome, if difficult, task.

Pharmacology or the study of how drugs affect animals and man (as opposed to the more familiar, pharmacy, which involves preparing and dispensing medicines) has until recently been restricted to schools of medical sciences. Few courses on pharmacology could be found at college level and the public's interest was very low. Several factors appear to have changed all that. Among these have been several highly-publicized, drug-related tragedies: the thalidomide infants, blood clots caused by widely used oral contraceptives (the "pill"), and, more recently, vaginal tumors in teenage women related to the hormone diethylstilbestrol (DES) given to their mothers to prevent miscarriage.

Another event that brought the word drug to the public consciousness was the "hippie" movement, which was associated with the psychedelic drugs. Slightly later, there was the sudden growth in hard street drugs and the abuse of amphetamines, heroin and "downers" which include barbiturates and other tranquilizers.

Interestingly, the past decade or so has also seen a rise in the number of prescriptions per capita in the United States of roughly the same magnitude as the rise in health care costs. Probably the two best-known medicines, Valium and Librium, appeared in the early 1960s and within a decade were in occasional use in an estimated 7%–10% of U.S. and European homes.

On the heels of these events came the rise of the U.S. consumer movement, lately including medical care. A wide array of books, pamphlets, and manuals on obtaining and maintaining good health within and without the traditional medical system has been produced, mostly well-intentioned.

Recently there have been demands for patient package leaflets for all medicines. This package "insert" will soon be available for some drugs, but the growing interest of drug consumers makes it probable that some day all patients will be provided information comparable to that available to their physician. In the long run, this may allow for joint decisions between patients and doctors on the proper medication.

But that day is in the future. This guide starts out by providing full, independent information now. It is based on the concept that an informed patient can obtain better medical care in the traditional medical system. It is hoped this information will encourage a better relationship and a dialogue with the physician to improve the patient's overall medical care and avoid problems. This can be particularly helpful when medication must be taken for long periods, or for several illnesses simultaneously, when risk benefit considerations become complex.

So this book has two major goals. Firstly to provide general information on drugs: how, why, and when they are used in general and in specific ailments. Secondly to spell out in an easily understood way detailed information about the most commonly prescribed drugs, including the therapeutic actions, possible adverse effects and interactions.

Part I – the Introduction – describes what drugs are in general, where they come from, how they work in the body and why they cause changes, lead to side effects and interact with other medication, food and drink. This will explain many words and ideas mentioned in later sections, and so it should at least be quickly skimmed to familiarize yourself with the subject before getting down to specifics.

Part II considers drugs according to the conditions for which they are most frequently used, looking at how certain ailments, such as high blood pressure, or diabetes, or asthma, are treated with the help of drugs. This part explains why certain drugs are used and how individual drugs relieve the symptoms of, or cure, a disease. Frequently doctors will change one specific drug used to treat a disease, for a different, but probably related, drug. This part will help you to understand the broader view of treatment, and provide an insight into how your doctor is thinking about the medicines he's giving you to take.

Part III is an alphabetical listing of the 200 most prescribed drugs, as well as some other commonly used medications and several newly introduced drugs. Medicines are listed in alphabetical order, either by their trade or brand name or by their generic name. Therefore, you can find a drug by using either the manufacturer's name or the internationally-recognized generic name. Each drug description gives you other brand names for the drug, the actions, side effects, precautions and interactions. Each drug is cross-referenced to the chapter in Part II which discusses that class of drugs in general, and gives you other background information.

For example, if you want to look up the drug *digoxin*, the drug will be found under that name (a generic name) with the trade name Lanoxin below. Following that are the action, dosage, adverse effects and interactions, and finally you are referred to the section on Drugs for Heart Failure.

Since it was impossible to list every drug that might be prescribed – there are many thousands available in the U.S. – many drugs other than those described are included in discussions of specific illnesses. Frequently, the medicine will be very similar to others in the group so the same general description often applies, but you should check in a recognized reference book, at most libraries, for more specific information.

It is hoped that this guide will be a useful source of information not only about the specific drugs, but also about the general diseases treated.

JUDITH K. JONES, M.D., PhD.
San Francisco, California

Part I   Introduction

What are drugs?
The world of drugs and medicines is considerably different from what it was 50 or 100 years ago. In the past, medicines were usually mixtures of many plant and mineral substances, prescribed in Latin by physicians and then deciphered and made up by pharmacists into elixirs, powders, or ointments that were often strange-smelling and tasting. Some of these unusual concoctions contained ingredients still seen in drugs today but many of the old medicines appear to have been effective as much through patients' expectations of good results as from anything else. (Nowadays we call this phenomenon a *placebo effect*, from the proven capacity of patients to benefit even from a harmless unmedicated preparation – a placebo – provided they believe it is a medicine that will do them good.)

The modern world of drugs and their regulation
Today we are in an entirely different era of drugs and medicines. Rarely are prescriptions written in Latin and rarely does the pharmacist himself prepare the mixtures except for some elixirs. Instead, most medicines are manufactured in large quantities, in the form of tablets, capsules, creams, suppositories and liquids (such as cough syrups or insulin) whose exact contents are carefully measured and standardized. Each type of drug, its production, distribution and availability, is now controlled by legislation that chiefly dates from the early- and mid-1900s, though new laws have been passed as recently as 1962.

Nowadays, before a drug can be introduced onto the market, it has to meet stringent standards of safety and effectiveness. To determine whether it does meet these requirements, it is first tested in many animals, and later in human volunteers and in persons with specific diseases.

These Food and Drug Administration requirements for safety and effectiveness have long been the subject of controversy. On the one hand, there is the real fear that another thalidomide (the sleeping pill which produced crippling birth defects in many children abroad) tragedy will occur if every drug is not carefully tested. On the other hand, such testing takes much time and delays introduction of many promising drugs. This has led to a frequently-expressed concern that the American public is being deprived of good, useful drugs, that are available in many other countries, because the Food and Drug Administration's requirements are too strict. There is no simple solution to this controversy.

Aspirin, and other drugs in use before the stricter laws governing the testing of drugs were passed, were not required to be tested as stringently due to a "grandfather clause" relating to their presumed safety as demonstrated by their many years of use.

Definitions of drugs and medicines
Drugs and medicines can be defined in terms of several characteristics – their use, their origins, and their actions, both helpful and harmful. In very general terms, a drug or medicine is any substance or mixture of substances which is used to improve people's physical or mental condition.

Sources of drugs
Drugs and medicines come from many different sources. In ancient times, "medicines" were made from extracts of plants, from certain animal materials, and occasionally, from mineral sources. In fact, many of our modern drugs are still derived from plants (for example, the quinine used for muscle cramps and quinidine used to control heart rhythm both come from the bark of the cinchona tree). Likewise, animal materials, such as the thyroid gland and the pancreas, are still the major sources of certain drugs such as thyroid and insulin. Minerals such as calcium and iron supplements still come from natural mineral sources. Since it was discovered that the simple bread mold produced the invaluable antibiotic penicillin, living fungi have been important sources of drugs – especially of antibiotics and the drugs used in cancer therapy.

Finally, some drugs such as Valium and Librium are chemically synthesized from organic chemicals – a major source of our medicines at present.

Drugs versus poisons
By definition, drugs are substances which are used to produce benefit, and poisons are substances which can, either intentionally or accidentally, cause harm. It is important to point out that any substance can in fact be either beneficial or poisonous depending on the dose taken, the intent of the individual taking it, and sometimes the presence or absence of disease in the person taking it.

For example, any drug taken in excessive amounts may be likely to cause adverse effects or poisoning. Conversely, some traditional poisons, such as curare, the poison used by South American Indians on their arrows, is a very useful drug in the controlled setting of a surgical operation. From another viewpoint, antibiotics often act as a "poison" to bacteria, but do not affect the host (ourselves). Similarly, many cancer drugs act as "poisons" to the tumor, and may also be somewhat toxic or "poisonous" to other organs, but are used because their overall benefit to a cancer patient is greater than the risk they entail.

Drug actions and "side effects"
Drugs can also be frequently defined or classified according to their actions. For example, a chemical which relieves pain, such as aspirin, is often classified as a pain reliever or analgesic, even though, like aspirin, it may be equally effective as a drug to relieve inflammation (anti-inflammatory) or to prevent clotting (anticoagulant). These actions may be seen as desirable effects in some cases (the relief of pain), and as "side effects" in other instances (when aspirin's anticoagulant effect is not desired). We have to consider drugs and medicines both from the point of view of their intended actions and uses, and from the point of view of their other, sometimes undesirable actions, or adverse effects.

How drugs act and interact
Drugs, if taken internally, can act on many organs, and sometimes alter their function. For example, certain drugs can adversely effect the functions of the kidney. Equally important, if two or more drugs are taken, there is sometimes a possibility of the two drugs interacting with each other. This can result in an increased, a decreased, or sometimes a wholly new effect from either or both of the drugs, and this is defined as a *drug interaction*. For example, when the anticoagulant drug Coumadin interacts with vitamin K in the liver, the two drugs cancel each other out. An interaction of this kind can be very significant for the health of the patient, and important drug interactions are noted at the end of each drug entry in the text.

The journey of a drug in the body
If a drug is swallowed, where does it go? It is useful to consider the journey of a drug through the body since this journey often determines how long the drug acts, and how strongly it acts. Once the drug is swallowed, it goes to the stomach, which often contains food, and almost always contains strong hydrochloric acid. Many drugs will begin to dissolve here, even before they pass along into the intestines and bowel. As they dissolve, they pass through the walls of the stomach, intestine and bowel and are carried out into the bloodstream directly to the liver. (Sometimes the presence of food or diarrhea can interfere temporarily with their absorption into the blood).

The liver is a type of processing "roundhouse" which processes all foods and chemicals so that they can be used or eliminated from the body. Through the long history of evolution, men and animals have developed a very sophisticated liver which can process the many complex chemicals present in plants and other foodstuffs. Some of the chemicals in the things we eat are toxic, and these the liver converts, by a process called *metabolism*, to less toxic substances which can be eliminated or used. Most drugs arriving at the liver are partly metabolized to other substances at this "first stop." Sometimes the metabolized drug is more, sometimes less, active than the original drug. Obviously, if the patient has a liver disease, like hepatitis, this metabolic function may be affected. This is why people with liver disease sometimes require lower doses of the drugs they take.

In the liver the drug can "hop onto" a carrier protein which will carry it around the bloodstream to the various organs, although some drugs will travel "freely" in the blood stream to all organs of the body. Once it reaches an organ it can attach to a protein molecule called a *receptor*, and at this point the action of the drug is seen. At the end of its journey, the drug is eliminated, usually via the bloodstream to the kidney to the urine. A good example of this can be seen if a person takes a multi-vitamin pill containing riboflavin. The vitamin will soon appear in the urine and make it yellowish-green. Occasionally drugs are also eliminated into the bile and therefore into the bowel. Obviously, if there is kidney failure, the drug cannot "leave" the body, and this accounts for the practice of using smaller doses or allowing longer intervals between doses of drugs to prevent accumulation.

When drugs are given by other methods – that is, intravenously, by injection, or in the form of suppositories – they enter the bloodstream directly and can go to the liver and therefore to the receptors. Some drugs, like creams and ointments, are for direct use on the skin and in the eye. These drugs usually do not go into the body, but they can if used in large amounts.

Frequency of dosing

What determines how often a drug must be taken? In earlier years it was generally felt that any drug was usually appropriately taken in divided doses (usually three or four times a day), a view based, in many cases, on the fact that the effect of the drug appeared to wear off in six to eight hours. More recently, however, two factors have changed this approach.

First, there is now a very popular trend towards measuring the amoung of the drug in the blood at various times. This has resulted in much closer scrutiny of drug effects and their length of action. It has also allowed a calculation of the drug's *half-life*. The half-life of a drug is the length of time it takes for the body to eliminate half the drug in the body. If a drug is given every half-life, relatively constant amounts of drug are present in the body. The major discovery of these studies was that many drugs which are frequently taken three of four times per day, such as Dilantin, allopurinol, and Elavil, have half-lives of longer than 24 hours and therefore could be taken only once daily and have a similar effect.

This development regarding a drug's half-life, has worked in support of a second popular trend: that of trying to make it easier for patients to follow the drug regimen prescribed by their physicians. It was found that patients who were required to take many pills a day tended either to forget or simply to refuse. This difficulty, defined as a problem in *compliance* or adherence to a prescribed regimen, can clearly be a serious one for the health of patients. Just as clearly, these patients would benefit from drug regimens that required less frequent doses of the medicines they need. As interest in the problem of patients' compliance has increased, so has the search for the drugs and drug dose forms which have longer actions and half-lives. This quest has already begun and is helping to improve therapy.

What determines dose?

The dose of a particular drug is usually standardized, although in fact there are often variable responses to the same amount of a drug. Dose sizes of drugs vary greatly – from grams, as in many antibiotics, to millionths of a gram as in the synthetic thyroid preparations. The effective dose of any drug is usually established by extensive testing – first on animals and then in humans.

It is important to note that the dose of any two drugs, even those with similar actions, should not necessarily be compared as to size or magnitude of effect. For example, 5mg (one thousandth of a gram equals one milligram) of Valium is often just as strong and effective a sedative as 100mg of phenobarbital. The dose of any particular drug only relates to the amount *of that particular* drug found to be effective.

Drugs in children
The prescribing of medicine for children presents certain problems, especially where infants are concerned, because their bodies' reaction to drugs tends to differ from adults'. For example, the liver, which metabolizes drugs in an adult body, may not be completely developed in an infant, and so cannot process drugs properly. In some cases this can lead to poisoning. Drugs can also have an opposite effect on children from the effect they have on adults. A classic example is the drug Ritalin, which is used to calm hyperactive children, while in adults it produces hyperactivity. These factors, plus the fact that the amount of drug needed to produce an effect in a child is much smaller, make the use of medicines in children a specialized subject. *Although some of the drugs prescribed in this book are also used to treat children, the doses for children are generally much lower than described here and are not specifically noted.*

Drugs in pregnant women
Since the thalidomide tragedy, there is a much greater and more widespread awareness of the potential danger of drugs taken during pregnancy, especially during the first eight to twelve weeks of pregnancy, when the development of vital fetal structures is taking place and can easily be adversely affected. Thalidomide, which was prescribed as a sedative, produced, when taken by the mother during this critical period, deformities in development of the arms and legs of unborn infants.

Unfortunately, partly because of the time-lag between the critical developmental period early in the pregnancy (often before pregnancy is discovered or even strongly suspected) and the birth of the infant, it has been difficult to identify the factors or drugs which have caused developmental problems in the fetus. Collecting exact information on the relationship between drugs and malformations also presents problems of various kinds. Animal studies, for example, do not relate specifically to what occurs in humans. Certain drugs can affect fetal development at only one critical time during pregnancy, but are otherwise not harmful. Other drugs are thought to be harmful throughout the pregnancy or for longer periods of time. For example, the antibiotic tetracycline can affect bone and teeth development and thus cannot be used in pregnancy at all and is contraindicated during most of childhood for the same reason. (Interestingly enough, tetracycline appears to cause ill-effects in the mother as well as in her unborn child).

The effects of excessive alcohol and cigarettes may also affect the developmental process in the fetus at several stages. But the adverse effects produced by alcohol and cigarettes seldom occur all of the time! In fact, even a drug which is known to cause specific effects may only cause those effects 5–20% of the time or even less. This may be because of the dose, the timing or other unknown factors. This makes the relationship between cause and effect very difficult to trace.

Still another problem is that the harmful effect of a drug taken during pregnancy may not be easily discovered for some period of time. This would be the case, for example, with adverse effects on intelligence or neurological development. A classic example of this type of problem is the DES or diethylstilbesterol problem. For a period of time, beginning in the mid-1940s, women who had a threatened miscarriage were given the hormone diethylstilbesterol to prevent this. Some 13 to 16 years later a small percentage of the female children born to these mothers had developed cancer of the vagina – a form of cancer that previously was very rare. Only very careful detective work on the part of pathologists who became suspicious about the increased rate of this rare cancer revealed the connection with DES. Not surprisingly, their discovery has increased the concern about drugs and pregnancy to an even greater extent. The state of knowledge about this subject will continue to be limited since adequate testing can frequently not be carried out. However, the general rule of obstetricians has been to have pregnant women avoid most drugs during pregnancy except vitamins, iron and a few other drugs which may be essential to the mother's health, such as thyroid hormone or insulin. However, the use of any drug during pregnancy is usually carefully supervised because of concern about the dangers.

The major problem still lies, not with women who are aware of their pregnancy, and are therefore more cautious, but with potentially-pregnant women who are taking drugs such as tetracycline, Valium or Librium which are now suspected of causing some birth defects in a small number of cases. Clearly, any woman of childbearing age who is currently having sexual relations and may become pregnant must exercise great caution where drugs and medicines of all kinds are concerned.

Drugs in the elderly

The third group who may have special responses to drugs are the elderly. Just who belongs in this classification is a moot point, since physiological ageing does not necessarily relate in any exact way to age in years. Nonetheless, when physiological ageing becomes apparent, it is often associated with changes in response to some drugs. One factor that contributes to this change is the gradual decline in the efficiency of the kidney in eliminating wastes (and therefore drugs). This is one of the reasons for the need to use lower doses of some drugs in elderly people. Since this change does not take place at the same rate in everyone, individual dosage adjustment may often be called for.

The use of various sedative and tranquilizing drugs – such as chloral hydrate, Seconal, Valium, Librium and Dalmane – by elderly people can be problematic for two reasons. First, as noted above, smaller doses may be needed, especially if regular use is planned, since the drug may accumulate and cause excess drowsiness. Secondly, some elderly persons, like children, may experience excitation rather than sedation with some of these drugs. The reason for this is not known, but it can cause confusion since often the response is to give more sedative!

Genetic factors

Genetic differences between people can also influence a drug's effect. For example, some individuals are more sensitive than others to small doses of the tricyclic antidepressant drugs, such as Elavil, Tofranil and Sinequan. Studies of those drugs showed that equal doses to several people would result in different levels of drug in their blood. However, identical twins had very similar blood levels. This suggested that at least some of the differences in blood levels were due to genetic factors in dealing with the drug in the body. The genetic causes of variable drug effects are only just beginning to be studied and defined at present, but in the future they may become well-accepted factors in determining the exact drug dose administered to each individual. Some individuals have genetic traits which can make common drugs harmful, though fortunately this is a relatively rare occurrence. People with the rare metabolic disease porphyria, for example, cannot take phenobarbital and certain related drugs because of the severe adverse reactions these drugs produce in them. Likewise, approximately 13% of the black population and a certain percentage of persons of Mediterranean origin have a deficiency of a certain enzyme in their red blood cells which makes them particularly susceptible to drugs used to treat malaria (primaquine), some sulfa drugs, and the drugs Furadantin and Macrodantin used to treat bladder and kidney infections. When any of these drugs are taken by persons with this enzyme deficiency, their blood cells begin to break down and they may develop fever and generalized discomfort. Fortunately, the presence of this enzyme deficiency can be detected by a simple blood test and the problematic drugs avoided. In many other cases, the genetic differences which cause these special effects cannot be anticipated. Further research into the problem may increase the chances of doing so in the near future.

Placebo effects

Another factor which strongly influences the way in which a drug will affect a person is the so-called *placebo effect*. In Latin, the work placebo means "I will please." In medical terminology, the word refers to a pill or other treatment which by itself has no chemical activity or drug-like effects on the body. (Frequently it is simply a pill made of sugar or lactose). However, when a placebo is given, it may in fact bring about certain changes in a patient's condition simply because the patient, or the doctor, or both, expect it to cause a change. These changes are called placebo effects. Placebos are most often used in studies of drugs to ascertain the effects of the real drug. This is very important since many people have marked responses to placebos. For example, most mild pain relieving drugs are tested against a placebo (in a double-blind test where neither the patient or the doctor knows which is the real drug) for the ability to relieve mild pain. Frequently, 20-40% of people receiving the placebo will experience pain relief! Further, if the study is geared to checking for side effects, it is frequently found that people may experience nausea, vomiting, itching of the skin or even rashes and other effects after taking the placebo. This is why the placebo effects of taking a drug must be subtracted from the final result of a drug test to determine the actual pharmacologic effect of the drug.

Why do people experience effects from a placebo? The reason lies in the *expectations* both of the person *and* of the therapist. For example, if a person has a headache and takes a pill which he expects will relieve his headache, he frequently will experience relief, even if the pill is completely inactive (a placebo). If this expectation of relief is enhanced by the enthusiastic expectation of effect by the doctor prescribing the pill, it is even more likely to achieve relief.

The placebo effect tends to be particularly noticeable in connection with drugs used for pain, sedation, tranquilization or other consciously-experienced sensations. It is very much less noticeable when the anticipated effect is not directly perceived, as in the case of antibiotics or heart medication.

Sometimes placebo drugs are administered when the physician feels that relief (often of mild anxiety) may be obtained as readily by the placebo effect of anticipated relief as by an active (and possibly harmful) drug. This is sometimes effective and is often done to protect the patient from chronic use of sedatives or pain relievers, not to "fool" the patient.

Effects of disease on drug effects
The effect of any given drug also varies in the presence of disease. For example, if a person has a fever, both aspirin and Tylenol will tend to bring the fever back down to normal, but in a person with normal temperature, these drugs will not significantly lower the body temperature. In a person suffering from a disordered perception of reality, as in schizophrenia, the use of phenothiazine drugs such as Thorazine will tend to normalize the thinking process, but the same drug will not markedly affect the thinking of a person in touch with reality. Other diseases simply change the way a drug is absorbed or metabolized or excreted. Thus, a person with severe diarrhea might not absorb much of a drug taken orally. A person with kidney failure may be unable to eliminate certain drugs, so they must be used in lower doses or less frequently lest they build up in his system.

Drug reactions
There is considerable public and medical concern over the side effects and adverse reactions to drugs. It is contended by some that drug reactions are a significant cause of hospitalization and of problems during hospitalization and various frightening statistics have been cited in the popular press.

However, some of the figures have represented general conclusions drawn from small studies and whether these are really accurate has been questioned. One recent large study of drug reactions in eight hospitals over a period of several years indicated that the rate of adverse reactions was not as high as previously thought. The controversy nevertheless continues.

Several points about drug reactions should be borne in mind when considering the problem:

1) Any drug is likely to have effects on many parts of the body. Some of these effects are desired, some are of little consequence, and some are not desired and are usually termed side or adverse effects. A side effect in one setting, such as the tendency of aspirin to inhibit blood clotting when it is used for arthritis, may be the desired effect when it is used in another setting, for example to prevent stroke.
2) Unwanted reactions to drugs fall into two main categories:
a) First are the known side effects of the drug, which can be anticipated and either accepted, prevented or treated. For example, the potassium loss that is a side

effect of taking a strong diuretic ("water pill") such as Lasix, can be prevented by adding potassium to the diet.

b) The second type of side effects are not as predictable, since they occur in only a small percentage of persons receiving the drug. They can be true allergic reactions, such as the rashes some people develop in response to penicillin. Or they can be the so-called "idiosyncratic" reactions, which are probably not allergic in nature but are rather related to the distinct genetic makeup of individuals and the way their particular bodies handle the drug. This latter type of reaction is much more difficult to anticipate or predict, since it may occur in only one out of 10,000 or 100,000 persons and may not be discovered before the drug is released for use. In contrast to the first caregory of reactions, these unwanted reactions cannot necessarily be prevented, but their possible occurrence is usually noted and considered in the cost-benefit analysis of the prescribing of any drug.

3) Very few drugs are free of unwanted side effects. Fewer still are free of the possibility of unpredictable allergic or idiosyncratic reactions. Some drugs have a greater potential for producing side effects than others. Thus, the prescribing of the drug by a physician usually is the result of a careful calculation of the benefits to the patient (i.e., relief in symptoms or curing the disease) versus the risks and cost to the patient. This consideration is closely related to the seriousness of the disease and the seriousness and frequency of the side effects. It is never a simple calculation. For example, in the treatment of arthritis, the benefits of higher-dose aspirin (effective relief of pain and inflammation at a relatively low cost), must be weighed against its disadvantages and risks (frequent dosing, hearing disturbances, gastric upset, bleeding or ulceration). A more difficult calculation is called for with the anti-cancer drugs; in this case, the possibility of their prolonging life must be weighed against their often very serious side effects, the need they entail for frequent and costly medical supervision, and sometimes, their very high cost.

Clearly, the decision as to whether the benefits of taking a drug outweigh the risks can be very difficult, and the problem is often complicated by a lack of sufficient information about the likelihood of side effects.

4) Certain conditions seem to increase the likelihood of drug reactions. The longer a drug is taken, for example, the more likely it is to cause side effects. Likewise, a higher dose of the drug may cause more side effects than a lower dose. A person who has already had allergic reactions (rashes, swelling of various areas of the body, or anaphylactic shock and wheezing) to one or more drugs is more likely to have an allergic reaction to another drug, particularly if that one is chemically related to the drugs that have produced allergic reactions in the past. It is important to note, however, that in most cases, nausea or vomiting after taking a drug (as for example, after taking codeine, Demerol or morphine) seldom represents a true allergic reaction, but rather an increased sensitivity to one of the known and expected effects of the drug.

Finally, the greater number of drugs a person takes, the more likely he is to experience side effects, not only because the individual effects of multiple drugs add up, but also because with several drugs, there is a greatly increased possibility of drug interactions.

Pinning down what is, and what is not, a genuine reaction to any one drug is not always easy. Just because a symptom occurs after taking a drug does not necessarily mean the drug caused that symptom. It may, for example, represent a placebo side effect or a totally separate problem. On the other hand, it sometimes happens that a side effect, such as headache or nausea, is ascribed to the underlying disease, while the drug as a cause is missed. In such cases, a simple discussion with a physician about whether a particular sign or symptom could be caused by a drug might clarify the situation early on, and save valuable time and discomfort for the patient.

Indeed, when a side effect is suspected, the doctor should always be consulted. In some cases, the drug will be stopped, not only to prevent further reaction, but also as a test to see if the effect goes away. In other cases, the side effect may be treated directly, as when antacids are given during treatment with aspirin or cortisone or prednisone to prevent the gastric irritation that is so often a side effect of these drugs.

Avoiding drug reactions

In general, it is a good rule for each individual not only to be aware of, but also to carry a list of those drugs which he or she is taking or those which have caused reactions. In our highly mobile society, visits to unfamiliar clinics, doctors or emergency rooms are a frequent occurrence, and specific information about a patient's drug history is often very helpful before treatment is given. A simple drug-information card can be made from a three by five card and carried in a prominent place in your wallet. An alternate plan is to use a metal bracelet or necklace which carries this information. The physician can often help in providing the relevant information.

The cost of drugs
Many drugs today are fairly expensive. Some people, in fact, have to pay a dollar a day or more for their drugs, and when these drugs must be taken over a period of months or years, the daily expense can add up to a heavy financial burden.

What determines the cost of a drug? In general, the cost of a drug to the patient is based on the costs of research and development, manufacture, advertising, packaging, shipping and pharmacy handling. But the price of an individual drug is not necessarily related to any of these factors.

Generic and brand name
Most drugs begin life as a basic chemical substance (such as penicillin, tetracycline or prednisone) which is produced by several manufacturers. These companies then sell them (in the form of tablets, capsules, ointments, etc.) directly to pharmacists or hospitals under generally accepted, less technical chemical names – their *generic* names. Alternatively, the manufacturers may apply *trade* or *brand* names to their products to differentiate them from the same products manufactured by other companies. Thus, tetracycline may be sold by its generic name, tetracycline hydrochloride, or by one of its trade names, such as Achromycin. Some manufacturers sell only generic products, both to pharmacists and to other companies, which apply their own brand names. Other drug manufacturers only sell their products under a trade name, though it may be available by a generic name from another manufacturer.

Frequently drugs are developed by one company and then produced and manufactured by that company under a drug patent which gives it exclusive rights to make and market the drug for 17 years. Once the 17 years have elapsed, the particular company holding the patent no longer has exclusive rights to the drug, so it may be produced and manufactured under its generic name as well as under new trade names. A good example in point is the drug Librium, whose patent has now expired and which is available under its generic name, chlordiazepoxide. In the case of many generic drugs, there are three or more companies selling the drug under different trade names. Thus, tetracycline hydrochloride is available under that generic name *or* as Achromycin, Robitet, SK-Tetracycline, and Retet. Ampicillin (the generic name) is available under that name as well as under the brand names Supen, Amcill, Omnipen, Polycillin, Pen-syn, Pen A, Penbritin and Principen. This multiplicity of brand names for one generic drug creates confusion on the part both of the prescribing doctor and his patient, but the drug industry argues that it allows for healthy competition on the drug market. It is doubtful, therefore, that the situation will change, although the rate of generic prescribing has been observed to be increasing.

A company will usually spend some money in promoting their brand-name product and this cost is usually added on to the basic cost of the drug. This means that, in general, trade-name drugs are more expensive (sometimes by several times) than their generic equivalent. This being so, many consumer groups have advocated that generic drugs be used in preference to brand-name drugs. There are, however, several factors which complicate this straightforward approach to the problem of high-cost brand-name drugs. First, many companies with brand-name products have argued that their drugs are more carefully tested and regulated than their generic equivalents. Indeed, it has been found that several products containing the same generic drug may be absorbed very differently, so that one may produce definite effects and another none at all. This has raised the entire issue of *bio-availability* (how much of the drug can be absorbed by the body to produce an effect), and led to stricter requirements on the part of the Food and Drug Administration for each manufacturer to prove that its drug is as bio-avialable as equivalent drugs.

In the long run, the drug companies' argument that their brand-name products represent better quality-control may tend to counteract generic prescribing. Many drug companies have also implied that their long-standing reputation as manufacturers of quality drugs is some basis for continuing to choose their products. Unfortunately, this generalization about quality may or may not apply, as almost every drug company has been subject to drug recalls and manufacturing problems at some point in its history.

Another factor which has confused the issue has been the "generic substitution" laws passed in many states. These regulations allow pharmacists to substitute one brand of a generic drug for another if the pharmacist deems this necessary for reason of better quality, lower price or stock supply. Thus, a prescription for erythromycin tablets in 250mg strength might be filled with large red, round tablets (Ilotycin), large, blue-green tablets (Robimycin) or large peach-colored tablets (E-Mycin), or a variety of other products. Any would contain the prescribed amount of erythromycin and the effect would in all probability be the same.

If the physician simply wrote the brand name on the prescription, any equivalent erythromycin could be substituted for it at the pharmacist's discretion. If, however, the physician also wrote "no substitution," on the prescription, the pharmacist would be required to fill the prescription with the particular brand of erythromycin specified by the physician, even if it cost considerably more. Sometimes a physician has a very definite reason for prescribing a brand-name product (as for example, to avoid confusion in the case of a patient taking several drugs) and sometimes not. It is often worth discussing the matter with the physician, because when there is no special reason for prescribing a brand-name drug, a switch to a generic prescription may save the patient money.

The cost of a drug, whether it is a generic or a brand-name product, can vary considerably depending on several factors. Prescriptions for large numbers of pills or capsules are usually less expensive, partly because medicines are packaged in larger lots and can be dispensed more easily. Also, each prescription does include a handling fee for the pharmacist, so that the more prescriptions needed by an individual patient, the more handling fees he or she must pay. Although smaller, private pharmacies tend to have somewhat higher prescription prices than larger chainstore operations, this is by no means always the case. Private pharmacies may also offer certain convenient extra services such as home delivery, drug profiles, counseling on the effects of the drugs, and so forth. Many states require that pharmacies post their drug prices so that persons who take drugs over long periods of time (such as persons with high blood pressure) may check prices at various sources and even report their findings back to their physician if they wish.

Another factor which influences the cost of prescriptions only affects those people on government health plans such as Medicaid and Medi-Cal. These people are granted allowances for their prescriptions, provided that their drugs are on the list of drugs approved. If they are not on this list, the patients must either pay for their prescriptions themselves or obtain a special request justifying the use of their particular drug before qualifying for their allowance. Since a limited number of allowances is available, the size of individual prescriptions is usually larger, a factor which has created some problems where drug abuse is a possibility.

In summary, then, how does one get the best quality drug at the most reasonable cost? First, it is helpful to indicate to the doctor a preference for a generically-named drug in maximum quantity (100-200 pills is customary) if it must be used for long periods. This is based on the generally valid assumption that in most cases generic drugs *are* equivalent and *are* less expensive than their brand-name counterparts. The doctor may have objections – both to prescribing a generic equivalent and to prescribing in quantity – but it should generate a useful dialogue. There are, of course, good reasons for small prescriptions of sedatives and narcotics, for example.

Secondly, in addition to comparing prices at various pharmacies, it is wise to consider the quality of the service those pharmacies provide. A good pharmacist, whose thorough training equips him to provide useful information about differences between drugs and advice about over-the-counter products, may well be worth some extra charge.

In this book there has been no attempt to state the price of any drug, but each listing includes both the generic name and one or more trade names. Some drugs, because they are most frequently prescribed by the generic name (such as ampicillin) are listed under that name with the trade names following. Other drugs in the 200 Most Frequently Prescribed List are best known by their trade names but the *generic* name is also given. For identification, the trade names are always capitalized; the generic names are not, except in the individual listings in Part III.

Part II A Brief Introduction to the Different Types of Drugs

Drugs for the relief of pain and/or inflammation

Pain is often our first indication that something is wrong, but treating the pain can sometimes be sufficient therapy – and in some types of diseases is still the only therapy possible. Drugs to relieve various types of pain or discomfort can generally be grouped into three categories, which overlap somewhat:

the three types of pain drugs
  –drugs for moderate to severe pain, primarily narcotic drugs;
  –drugs for mild pain such as headache;
  –drugs which can relieve both pain and inflammation, usually of joints, as in the case of aspirin for arthritis.

Before considering these three drug groups, it will be helpful to review the whole subject of pain and the principles behind the methods used to relieve it.

what is pain?
Pain can be defined as the perception of discomfort due to irritation, chemical stimulation or stretching of a pain nerve ending. Pain nerves are located throughout the body, except inside the brain, and send signals indicating pain to the brain, where they are registered and perceived. The brain may then send return signals back to the body, usually to the muscles, initiating withdrawal from the pain. Prevention or relief of pain can thus be accomplished in several ways. We all know, for example, that the total perception of pain in major surgery can be eliminated by general anesthesia, which simply puts the perceptive organ (the brain) to sleep. Perception of very localized pain, of the kind experienced in dental work, can be similarly avoided by preventing the initiation of signals by pain nerves in the region through the use of local anesthetics such as procaine (Novocaine). In rare cases of chronic pain, the pain nerves themselves can be cut, usually near the spinal cord. These methods of preventing or relieving

special kinds of pain do not involve the drugs and medicines we normally use, and so are not discussed further in this book.

For most types of pain the means of relief in most cases is to remove or eliminate its cause, or, alternatively, to decrease the sufferer's perception of the pain. The pain of red, swollen, inflamed joints can be relieved in part by drugs that decrease the inflammation, such as aspirin. The perception of pain from an uninflamed joint, however, can only be relieved by a drug that changes a person's perception of what he describes as pain.

variations in pain

The subject of pain and its relief is a very complex matter because of the considerable variation of pain perception between individuals and the difficulty of objective measurement. For example, ask a few people to describe the pain of an ordinary heachache and the responses are likely to vary from "a dull ache," to "a sharp shooting pain," to a "band around the head," to many other descriptions – try it sometime. Why the variation? One reason is that the cause of headache pain actually varies from muscle spasm, to injury, hangover, sinisitus, eye fatigue, to a true migraine headache. In turn, differing sources may affect the *quality* of the pain, sharp vs. dull for example. Another reason has to do with the duration of the pain. What begins as a relatively sharp headache pain (and is newly perceived) may take on a dull, throbbing character as the headache persists.

psychological factors

An important additional reason relates to the many psychological factors which affect the *perception* of pain. These include learned or cultural, and perhaps even genetic or inherited influences. They also include the emotional impact of the pain (if the pain raises the question of cancer or a heart attack it will always be very noticeable until the suspicions are disproved), and they include the presence or absence of other distracting factors, as when we suddenly dismiss a headache at the beginning of a long-awaited party. Just as the pain is influenced by all these factors, so will the effects of any drug designed to change perception of the pain. And, of course, the effectiveness of any such drug is partly dependent upon the *expectations* of the person taking it and of the doctor prescribing it. A tablet or capsule that someone strongly believes will work will be effective more frequently, even if it is really only a sugar pill (a *placebo*, with no chemical effect) than a pill believed to be useless in the first place.

This placebo effect, which is owing to expectation rather than to the true chemical or pharmacologic effect on the body, often leads doctors to prescribe sugar pills to "cure" non-existent diseases. It is a very powerful phenomenon, as demonstrated by tests showing that 30 – 40% of people with mild pain will get relief from a sugar pill if they believe it is a pain killer. This factor makes the evaluation of pain medicines, in fact all medicines, fairly difficult, especially when only mild pain or symptoms are involved.

controlling pain
perception

Most drugs for relief of pain primarily alter perception and are called, as a group, *analgesics*. They can be divided into drugs for severe pain, and drugs for mild pain. Some of the latter drugs also help relieve one cause of pain – inflammation – and are considered separately, later.

Acute (temporary) and chronic (continuous and recurring) pain are often perceived in different ways. The drugs that relieve pain also act in more than one way, with the possible exception of local anesthetics, which simply temporarily "deaden" the nerve carrying pain signals to the brain. Most pain medications act primarily to decrease perception of the pain, although some, especially aspirin and related anti-inflammatory drugs, also act locally at the site of the pain.

Narcotic analgesics (see separate chapter) primarily decrease perception of pain, often by producing a transient feeling of well-being or euphoria. Non-narcotic analgesics (see separate chapter) also decrease perception of pain, acting both near the site of pain and on the brain. They are less potent than narcotics, and are not generally addictive, at least physically.

Those analgesics that also have anti-inflammatory properties (see Drugs for the Relief of Pain and or Inflammation; Drugs for Pain with Inflammation) usually have more side effects, particularly gastrointestinal upset. Frequently these analgesics are formulated as combinations of aspirin, phenacetin and caffeine with or without other analgesics such as codeine (a narcotic), and Darvon (propoxyphene). The relative usefulness of these combinations is discussed under the individual products. In general the actual function of caffeine in these drugs is unknown and the use of phenacetin, which may cause kidney damage with long term use, has been challenged, and in some countries discontinued.

Two recent research breakthroughs hold out the hope of even more effective, and better-controlled methods of treating pain. One is the notion of a central biasing mechanism a sort of "gate-control," in the brain that can affect the perception of pain. Researches believe that stimulating the mechanism that controls pain "feeling" can effectively shut the gate to pain sensations. In part, this helps explain the usefulness of electrical stimulation therapy and acupuncture, as well as age-old "natural" remedies for pain such as hot cups, ice packs and even mudpacks.

The other research discovery is that the human body itself produces its own natural potent pain-relievers, called enkephalins (meaning "in the head"). Once these substances were identified, it was hoped that by chemical synthesis useful non-narcotic non-addictive pain-relievers could be produced. Thus far this has not been successful but it offers a hopeful area in researching new drugs for pain.

But taken together, these two steps have given scientists new paths to follow in their search for better medicaments for the treatment of all types of pain.

Narcotic pain relievers

Most of the drugs used for severe pain are considered narcotics and are related to morphine. All of these drugs act to decrease perception of pain and tend to produce a temporary sense of well-being or euphoria. This in part accounts for the abuse of these drugs, even those under the supervision of a physician.

narcotic drug dependence and addiction

When used repeatedly and regularly for many days or weeks, the dose of narcotic drug needed to effectively relieve pain or cause a feeling of well-being must be increased owing to the development of tolerance to the drug. If the narcotic is suddenly discontinued, withdrawal symptoms, such as marked nervousness or stomach cramps, may occur, indicating physical dependence upon the drug. These symptoms are rapidly relieved when the drug is taken and thus a cycle can develop in which it is difficult to permanently discontinue the drug. The presence of tolerance and physical dependence are indications of "addiction" to the narcotic.

Despite the hazard of addiction, the potent narcotic analgesics remain highly valuable drugs when used carefully and only when needed for relief of severe pain. Because of the addiction potential, however, this class of medication is restricted in its use and distribution in hospitals and pharmacies, according to regulations established by the U.S. Drug Enforcement Agency.

Listed below are some of the commonly prescribed narcotic pain relievers. Those with an asterisk are individually described in Part III.

A.S.A. Compound	Fiorinal with	Synalgos-DC*
codeine*	codeine*	Tylenol with
Demerol*	morphine*	codeine*
Dilaudid	Percodan*	
Empirin Compound	Phenanphen with codeine*	
with codeine*		

Non-narcotic pain relievers

Although a very large number of products for relief of mild-to-moderate pain are available on both the over-the-counter and prescription drug market, it is important to point out that they are generally composed of one or more of three basic components, all of which can relieve mild pain: aspirin, acetaminophen, and phenacetin (which is converted to acetaminophen) or the Darvon group of drugs. These are often combined with each other or with small amounts of the mild stimulant caffeine and sometimes smaller amounts of codeine or tranquilizers. Frequently the drugs are essentially equivalent except for their cost and packaging, although it can even be reasonably argued that both of these latter factors increase the expectation of greater effect!

Listed below are some of the commonly prescribed non-narcotic pain relievers and muscle relaxants. Those with an asterisk are individually described in Part III.

Non-Narcotic pain relievers:	Darvon Compound-65*	
	Equagesic*	
acetaminophen*	Fiorinal*	**Muscle relaxants:**
aspirin*	Norgesic*	Parafon-Forte*
Darvocet-N*	Talwin*	Robaxin-750*
Darvon*	Tylenol*	Soma Compound

Drugs for pain with inflammation

The word inflammation is a general term which applies to the occurrence of swelling, along with pain and often external redness. Inflammation is a very complex response of the body to various noxious stimuli such as insect stings, local infections, or abscesses such as boils, injury such as a broken bone or burn, and in chronic disease such as rheumatoid or gouty arthritis. In all of these, the area affected becomes red, swollen and painful. The treatment of inflammation often involves eliminating the cause through means other than medication, for example by draining an abscess or treating an infection.

arthritis and anti-inflammatory drugs

However, one type of inflammation is fairly consistently relieved by a group of drugs called anti-inflammatory drugs, and this includes a variety of inflammations of the joints called arthritis. The term arthritis applies to a group of diseases that affect the joints of the body causing chronic pain and often swelling, and eventual destruction of joints. Some types of arthritis are associated with acute inflammation (that is, swelling, redness and pain) of several joints. The most common of these "inflammatory" arthritis disorders are rheumatoid arthritis and gouty arthritis. Both of these diseases have courses which vary so that there are "flares" alternating with asymptomatic periods of normality. There are several drugs which are effective in treating the acute flares by slowing the inflammatory process and relieving pain, and sometimes even preventing their occurrence. The drugs effective in one disease (such as colchicine in acute gout) are not necessarily effective in the other, and sometimes their application is actually used by doctors as a kind of diagnostic aid, for example, if colchicine doesn't work, then it's probably not gout.

A very common type of arthritis, called osteoarthritis, is associated with little inflammation, but can cause tenderness of many, especially large, joints. Pain of a chronic nature is a greater problem here than inflammation. This type of arthritis can often be treated with pain-relievers with no anti-inflammatory effect, such as acetaminophen.

The drugs used for arthritic pain generally have the property of causing a slow-down of the inflammatory process, although they do this in diverse ways. Somewhat unfortunately, most of the drugs that have this anti-inflammatory effect also share the tendency to promote ulceration or irritation of the stomach. Except for aspirin, most of these drugs tend to relieve pain more by helping to relieve the inflammation causing the pain than by changing perception of the pain. Several new anti-inflammatory drugs have recently been put on the market and the most widely used, Motrin, is discussed in Section III. Although these drugs have been shown in short-term studies to be equal in effectiveness to aspirin in relief of chronic arthritic pain, they are far more costly and share many of the side effects of aspirin and the other anti-inflammatory drugs.

Listed below are some of the commonly prescribed anti-inflammatory drugs. Those with an asterisk are individually described in Part III.

aspirin*	Indocin*	Naprosyn
Butazolidin	Nalfon	Tandearil*
Butazolidin Alka*	Motrin*	Tolectin

Drugs for treating sleep disorders and problems with anxiety, mood or thought

Medication used for treating anxiety, mood, sleep or thought disorders makes up the most commonly prescribed group of drugs. Although sedative and tranquilizing substances (not the least of which is alcohol) have been used for centuries, it is only in the last 20 years that a range of drugs for treating nervous disorders has become available. Development of more sophisticated drugs in this area has broadened the types of problems treatable with medication, although the origins of many of these disorders and the mode of action of the drugs themselves remain mysterious.

Drugs in this category fall into two major classes:
1) Those used for mild, self-limited problems that are part of the ordinary stresses of life, such as sedatives or tranquilizers for anxiety, and sleeping pills for the occasional disturbance of normal sleep patterns.
2) Those used for more disrupting disturbances that seriously interfere with day-to-day behavior, such as the major tranquilizers for thought disorders and the antidepressants and lithium for disabling problems of mood.

A group of drugs called stimulants is usually used in problems with weight control, so they are more thoroughly discussed in the chapter on that subject.

Minor tranquilizers

popularity of
tranquilizers

Minor tranquilizers, also called anti-anxiety agents, are part of the most frequently prescribed drug group, along

25

with sleeping pills. In fact the leading minor tranquilizer, Valium, is the most prescribed medicine in the United States. Since the introduction of Librium and Valium the percentage of the population taking such medication has sharply increased, reflecting promotional efforts to physicians, increased access to health care, and possibly, heightened environmental stress.

Minor tranquilizers, sleeping pills and sedatives have very similar effects – their differences are more related to dosage and or prescribing pattern than to pharmacological activity. For example, Dalmane, which is used most often for sleep, is not significantly different from Valium, Librium, Serax or Tranxone, which are usually prescribed as anti-anxiety agents. Similar anti-anxiety drugs include barbiturates such as phenobarbital, antihistamines such as Vistaril or Atarax, and drugs such as meprobamate.

success of benzodiazepines

But the first group (Librium, Valium, Serax and Tranxene), known as benzodiazepines, is by far the most commonly taken. The major difference between tranquilizers and sleeping pills is their potential for (1) abuse, (2) death when taken in overdose, and (3) drug interactions. The benzodiazepines appear to have the lowest potential for all these problems. However, the barbiturate group, including phenobarbital and Seconal, as well as Quaalude and Doriden (which are more commonly used as sleeping pills) have high potentials for all of these and require very judicious use.

antihistamines as tranquilizers

Another group of drugs, the antihistamines, has significant sedative effects in certain individuals, although their actions differ from other drugs in this group (see Antihistamines). Since they are relatively safe, antihistamines are often used both as tranquilizers and sleeping pills; they have long been major components of over-the-counter sleep preparations.

dosage variation

All of these drugs lower anxiety and often allow a calmer, though altered, perception of life at "tranquilizing" doses. The effect of any drug dose appears to vary among individuals, in tranquilizers as in most medication. For example, 5 mg of Valium (the usual anti-anxiety dose) may calm one person, put another to sleep, make a third feel dizzy, and have no effect on a fourth. Occasionally, these drugs can actually excite – especially children or the elderly – but most people are tranquilized at this dose. At higher doses, especially when taken at night, these drugs can help induce sleep, though the sleep is different from unassisted sleep and with habitual use, real sleeping and dreaming time may decrease, an effect discussed in detail in the next section on sleeping pills.

The major side effect in using minor tranquilizers is drowsiness, which is often a function of dose. Of course this can be a useful effect if the drug is used at night. A very small percentage of persons taking these drugs also experience confusion, disorientation or even vertigo.

not without
hazards

All these drugs share characteristics which can make them hazardous in certain situations:

(1) they can depress breathing in persons with significant lung disease or when taken in excessive dosage; (2) they are additive to one another and to alcohol in producing sedation or sleep and in depressing breathing (this explains some accidental deaths due to intake of slightly excessive amounts of sedatives with alcohol); (3) they can be habit-forming. Once a habit is established, not only is it difficult to stop, but withdrawal symptoms can follow sudden drug-stoppage. In mild cases this may only mean nightmares or some anxiety for several days. In more severe cases, seizures can result.

Mild tranquilizers are often prescribed for use two to four times a day, but in many cases this may be excessive, or unnecessary. Firstly, anxiety is often transient and may require only occasional doses rather than continuous use. Secondly, drugs like Valium, Librium and phenobarbital stay in the body for long periods, so often they can be taken just once a day.

Listed below are some of the commonly prescribed minor tranquilizers. Those with an asterisk are individually described in Part III.

Atarax*	meprobamate*	Tranxene*
Equanil*	phenobarbital*	Valium*
Librium*	Serax*	Vistaril*

Sleeping pills

Most tranquilizers can be used as sleeping pills, and vice versa, as noted in the previous section. However, drugs such as chloral hydrate, Dalmane, Seconal and Nembutal are more commonly prescribed as sleeping pills, though in lower doses they have essentially the same effects as daytime tranquilizers.

routine use
effective?

Before some recent studies of sleep characteristics,

sleeping pills were routinely administered in hospitals and nursing homes, and frequently prescribed for use at home for treating common insomnia. But our greater understanding of the phenomenon we call sleep has cast doubt on the wisdom of using sleeping pills routinely. These studies of brain waves showed that normal sleep consists of several stages (numbered 0 to 4). After going to sleep, there is a stepwise descent from stage 0 to 4 then back and forth for three or more cycles. Dreaming usually occurs after return to stage 1, and since it is accompanied by eye movements, it is called rapid eye movement, or REM, sleep. REM sleep appears to be important, because anyone deprived of REM sleep for long periods may become irritable, anxious, or even begin hallucinating. It was also discovered that the majority of sleeping pills tend to change the normal sleep cycle. For example, barbiturates such as Seconal, Nembutal or Tuinal, or the drug Doriden, tend to suppress REM sleep. Drugs like Dalmane or low doses of chloral hydrate, do not affect REM sleep, but can eliminate stage 4 sleep. Studies on long-term users of sleeping pills indicate that not only do they skip REM sleep, but they tend to wake up several times during the night! The full meaning of these and other studies still needs to be clarified, but they do indicate that sleeping pills do not produce normal sleep. Because of this, most doctors have become more selective in prescribing sleeping pills, and caution should be exercised in using any non-prescription products to aid sleep.

abuse and suicide change outlook

Another factor prompting caution on the use of sleeping pills is the significant problem of abuse with many of these drugs, such as Seconal, Nembutal and Quaalude. The prescribing of many of these drugs has been restricted in a manner similar to that of narcotics. A third factor with sleeping pills is their use in suicide attempts, especially in certain age groups. The therapeutic approach to insomnia is changing, because, like pain, it is often a symptom of other physical or mental problems. Sometimes it reflects depression, and when this is addressed, sleep improves. Other times, insomnia may be a transient reaction to specific life stresses, and will disappear in its own good time. Although sleeping pills are still helpful in some situations for short-term assistance, their use should be more selective in the future.

Listed below are some of the commonly prescribed

sleeping pills. Those with an asterisk are individually described in Part III.

Butisol*	Nembutal*	Seconal
chloral hydrate*	Noludar	Tuinal
Dalmane*	Quaalude	
Doriden*	Placidyl*	

Major tranquilizers

The group of drugs called major tranquilizers, or anti-psychotic drugs, must not be confused with the more commonly used minor tranquilizers or anti-anxiety agents such as Librium or Valium, discussed in an earlier chapter. Major tranquilizers, although they have the ability to cause sedation, have a broader range of physiological effects and strong adverse reactions, so they are used only in special controlled situations for treating disorders of thinking.

True major tranquilizers came into being in the early 1950s, revolutionizing the care of severely disturbed patients. Using these drugs, called phenothiazines, enabled many persons previously confined to mental hospitals to return to a relatively normal life. This is because one of the major actions of these drugs is to return thinking processes toward normal. Frequently the effects can be dramatic in people with severe thought disorder who have hallucinations or loss of contact with reality, as in schizophrenia, or certain types of neurological diseases. Although the major tranquilizers do not always eliminate the need for other types of therapy, they have very wide usage. Often the most effective treatment for thought disorders involves a major tranquilizer in combination with psychiatric and/or social therapy.

These drugs are promoted and sometimes used for treating anxiety problems that do not involve disorders of thinking. Although the sedative effect of many of the major tranquilizers does help in these cases, it is very questionable whether such potent drugs are needed. Other actions of these drugs allow their use in different clinical settings. For example, one drug, Compazine, is primarily used to treat nausea.

wide variations in effects

Major tranquilizers work by acting on nerve endings in the brain and elsewhere in the body. There is wide variation in response to these drugs, and a correspondingly

29

large variation in the effective dose. Major tranquilizers stay in the body for a long time, so when used over extended periods, they are usually taken once daily, sometimes with no drug on weekends, to prevent accumulation. These drugs must be used selectively because of the wide variety of side effects, some of which are predictable, others not. The most common side effects are discussed here.

neurological effects

Almost all major tranquilizers can produce neurological effects, the most common being symptoms resembling Parkinson's disease, which is characterized by hand tremors, some rigidity of the arms and legs and a "mask-like" facial appearance. These symptoms can be overcome with a standard anti-Parkinsonian drug, such as Cogentin (see Drugs for Parkinson's Disease), without interrupting treatment, or by changing to a related neuroleptic. Other neurological effects are less predictable, such as grimacing of the face and twitching in the extremities. A marked withdrawal symptom after major tranquilizers are stopped is characterized by uncontrolled trembling and circular movement of the tongue and lips. This unpredictable effect, called "tardive dyskinesia" may be aggravated by antiParkinsonian drugs, although sometimes it improves with increased doses of the major tranquilizer. This effect is a principal reason why those drugs must be used quite selectively and with frequent medical checkups.

sedation

Many of these drugs produce mild sedation, particularly Thorazine and Mellaril. This effect is sometimes put to use by giving the daily dose at bedtime to avoid interference with daytime activities.

low blood pressure

Some of these drugs, again especially Thorazine and Mellaril, tend to produce low blood pressure. This effect tends to decrease with time, but when present, may produce dizziness when moving from a reclining to a sitting position. This is prevented by changing position slowly, or by switching to a related drug with less of this effect, such as Prolixin, Stelazine or Haldol.

anticholinergic effects

Like the antispasmodic drugs such as Pro-Banthine and the tricyclic antidepressant drugs such as Elavil, major tranquilizers block the substance acetylcholine produced by the nervous system. This substance controls many body functions and blockage may cause a dry mouth, difficulty with bladder function (especially in older persons), constipation, and changes in the eye, which can predispose to glaucoma. These effects may decrease with time, but can be increased if an antiParkinsonian drug, such as Cogentin, is used.

idiosyncratic effects

Certain adverse effects to these drugs are relatively rare. These include jaundice (yellow discoloration of the skin, eyes and urine) due to liver damage, a marked decrease in the white blood count (predisposing to severe infection), and various allergic reactions such as skin rash. These serious effects usually appear within the first few months and should be reported immediately. If allergy develops to one of the phenothiazine-type major tranquilizers, an agent with a different chemical structure, such as Haldol, is usually substituted.

One major tranquilizer is now combined with a tricyclic antidepressant (see following chapter), and the two products (Triavil, Etrafon) are frequently used in various types of depression of anxiety. For several reasons there is considerable question whether this combination has any appropriate use. The response to both types of drugs is highly variable and seldom can a fixed combination provide the proper dose of each. Furthermore, the anticholinergic effects of both drugs are additive, so, in most cases, one drug or the other is preferable.

Listed below are some of the commonly prescribed major tranquilizers and drugs that combine a major tranquilizer with an antidepressant. Those with an asterisk are individually described in Part III.

major tranquilizers	Stelazine*	drugs combining
Compazine*	Taractan	a major
Haldol	Thorazine*	tranquilizer and
Mellaril*	Trilafon	a tricyclic
Navane		antidepressant:
Prolixin		Etrafon*
Sparine		Triavil*

Antidepressants and lithium

depression and elation

Variations in mood from elation to depression occur normally to almost everyone. In some, the degree to which moods are felt may be exaggerated. When a person sees himself and his life in a wholly negative way the mood can lead to inability to work and occasionally to suicide. However, such a state is almost always temporary and after a time the mood lightens. In some the mood may lighten to the point of elation, which can be so excessive that a person thinks he can achieve things well beyond his means or capacity. While all of these moods are experienced occasionally, when a person has long-standing, repeated, excessive mood changes, it interferes with day-to-day activities and relationships, and therefore requires treatment. Recurrent depression is called unipolar endogenous depression, while fluctuations from depression to marked elation is called manic-depression, a bipolar state. Though serious, long-standing problems of mood are treatable with specific medication, these drugs are sometimes used inappropriately to treat minor mood problems, especially depression. Many life changes, such as the death of someone close, or even moving to an unfamiliar place, can cause depression. But unless there is a history of recurrent, serious depression, these passing episodes will usually improve by themselves or with supportive therapy – often before drugs used in recurrent mood disorders could take effect, which may be more than three weeks. Thus, problems that will truly be helped by antidepressant drugs are fairly specific.

Until the 1960s, the treatment of serious depression included use of stimulant drugs such as amphetamines (which when withdrawn cause even worse depression), electroshock therapy, and another class of drugs still in occasional use called, after their effect on an enzyme, monoamine oxidase (MAO) inhibitors. MAO inhibitors include the drugs Parnate and Nardil, which rarely are also used to treat high blood pressure. The MAO inhibitors are relatively effective in reversing depression, but are seldom used today due to drug interaction that can result in severe hypertension and sometimes stroke when they are taken with certain types of cheese, red wine and brewers yeast.

tricyclics replace
MAO inhibitors

Fortunately, a group of drugs related to medication for thought disorders (such as Thorazine) was introduced shortly after the MAO inhibitors. Called tricyclic antidepessants because of their chemical structure, they are the most useful drugs for serious depression and include: amitriptyline (Endep, Elavil), imipramine (Tofranil, Imavate, Janimine, Presamine, SK-Pramine), doxepin (Adapin, Sinequan), nortriptyline (Aventyl), and desipramine (Norpramine, Pertofrane).

A major difficulty with tricyclics is that they may take up to three weeks to take full effect. This problem is compounded by the fact that when first given, they have anticholinergic effects that can result in a very dry mouth, difficulty in urinating (especially if prostate trouble is present), sleepiness and blurred vision or constipation. In short, a person starting these drugs may actually feel worse, and must be strongly supported until they take effect. Luckily, at about the time the antidepressant effect takes hold, the side effects tend to become less bothersome.

The sedative effect of tricyclic antidepressants is often put to good use. As these drugs tend to stay in the body for more than a day or two, they often are taken at night when they can also promote sleep.

In addition to the temporary side effects noted above, tricyclics occasionally affect heart rhythm so their use in persons with heart disease requires careful observation.

serious drug interactions

Tricyclic antidepressants tend to have serious drug interactions with two types of drugs: the antihypertensive drug guanethidine (Ismelin), which is made less effective; and other anticholinergic drugs such as those for stomach spasm, gastrointestinal disorders and for Parkinsonian symptoms, where additive effects can cause marked constipation or bladder problems.

Two products (Triavil and Etrafon) combine the antidepressant amitriptyline (in Elavil and Endep) with the phenothiazine major tranquilizer perphenazine (Trilafon). Since the two disorders that the components of these combinations are used to treat usually require individualized doses, the likelihood that a fixed combination can be effective is very low.

Lithium compounds

When mood swings tend more toward marked elation, alternating with mild or severe depression, a mineral salt called lithium carbonate (Eskalith and Lithane) is extremely useful in allowing people to function normally. When using this preparation, however, dosage and blood level must be carefully monitored since excessive doses can be very dangerous.

Other drugs, such as the major tranquilizers or antidepressants, are sometimes used in treating this euphoric condition, but response is highly individualized.

Listed below are some of the commonly prescribed antidepressants and drugs that combine an antidepressant and a major tranquilizer. Those with an asterisk are individually described in Part III.

antidepressants:	Tofranil*	drugs combining
Aventyl	Vivactil	an antidepressant
Elavil*		and a major
Norpramine		tranquilizer:
Sinequan*		Etrafon*
		Triavil*

Drugs for heart and vascular disorders

Cardiovascular disease is a major cause of death and hospitalization and a principal contributor to the need for continued medical care in the United States. Thus, it is not surprising that many of the most frequently prescribed drugs come into the general classification of cardiovascular drugs, nor that these fall into a large number of categories.

As an introduction to looking at these important individual groups of drugs and what they do (discussed in separate chapters) it is necessary to consider briefly what the "cardiovascular system" is, how it works, and how drugs can affect it.

the work of the cardiovascular system

The term cardiovascular refers to the heart (cardiac), plus the associated blood vessels (vasculature), which include the arteries, the veins, and the tiny vessels that connect the arteries and veins, called capillaries. Under normal conditions, the cardiovascular system can be considered as a closed system of tubes (blood vessels), with a pump (heart) to move the blood through these tubes. The main purpose of the system is to deliver oxygen (which is picked up when the blood passes through the lungs) and other nutrients by way of the arteries to the capillaries, where the oxygen and nutrients pass across the capillary walls to the tissues. Further along, the capillaries become veins and the blood is returned, back to the lungs to pick up more oxygen and to the heart for another cycle. The ability of this system to give efficient blood flow to the tissues is not unlike that of a mechanical pump system and is related to the efficiency of the pump, the size and openness of the blood vessels or tubes, and the pressure in the system, which is a function of the strength of the heart contraction (heart beat) as well as the stiffness of the artery walls.

This system is very finely tuned, but flexible, so it is able to adapt quickly to many situations, such as exercise and stress. But if damage occurs to the system, either from disease or injury, there can be several problems, and different types of drugs must then be used to try and return the system to normality.

drugs for heart failure

If the heart is not getting enough oxygen due to clogged arteries serving the heart muscles (coronary arteries), the heart may not function as efficiently as it should or contract as well as it has in the past.

This turn of events may result in a signal to the kidneys to retain salt and water in order to keep the maximum amount of volume and pressure in the system. Although this maneuver helps, on a short term basis, to maintain blood flow and volume, it can also further stress the heart as it has more volume to pump and therefore more work to do. Because blood flow is less efficient, some of the retained salt and water goes out into the tissues to cause edema, or swelling of the tissue, especially in the lungs and the feet. This can result in a sensation of shortness of breath. The whole group of symptoms is called heart failure. In this condition, where the heart may not function at its peak, the type of medication most frequently given includes diuretics (see chapter on Diuretics), which promote loss of water and salt from the kidneys thus decreasing the volume in the cardiovascular system, and "easing the load" on the heart. The other usual drug for heart failure is one given to stimulate the heart, usually one of the digitalis drugs, like digoxin (see Drugs for Heart Failure). These drugs, called cardiac glycosides, increase the strength of the heart's contraction, improve the efficiency of action including the heart rate, and actually bolster the heart's ability to react normally to stimulation for additional output. 1984565

drugs to regulate the heart rhythm

This closed circulatory system also functions less efficiently if the heart (pump) beats irregularly or too rapidly so that all the blood in the heart may not be pumped out each time, which can also result in heart failure. Abnormal rhythm can decrease blood flow to the capillaries and the delivery of oxygen to the tissues. Therefore, many drugs that act on the electrical conduction system of the heart are used to make the heart rhythm slower and more regular (see Drugs for Abnormal Heart Rhythms) including digoxin or Lanoxin (which affects the heart rhythm as well as the strength of contraction), quinidine, Pronestyl and Xylocaine.

drugs for hypertension and angina pectoris

When the heart beats" (called systole) it must contract or pump against both the pressure of the astery walls and the volume of blood in the closed tube system. If the arteries are constricted, as if often true in a condition of increased blood pressure (hypertension), the heart must pump harder than normal to generate sufficient pressure to get blood to the tissues and other organs. If the heart is already weakened, the need to generate further pressure puts it under even greater strain. Some drugs are now being used to decrease this pressure (called "afterload") by opening up or relaxing the arterial blood vessels and therefore decreasing the work and strain on the heart. A secondary effect of these drugs is that they also improve blood flow to the heart, which can bring a decrease in angina pectoris (intermittent pain in the heart). The drugs used in this way include nitroglycerin, Isordil and a new class of medication called beta-blockers (see Drugs for Angina Pectoris).

drugs which decrease blood clotting

When the heart is functioning less efficiently, frequently the blood now in this closed system may be less efficient. Especially in the return system, made up of veins, this condition may predispose to sluggish flow and thus to blood clotting within the blood vessels, which is called thrombosis. There are also many other causes of thrombosis that do not directly relate to failure of the cardiovascular system. If clots which are formed travel to the lung through the veins, they can cause a "pulmonary embolus," which can affect the heart and the exchange of oxygen in the lungs. To prevent further formation of these clots, drugs called anticoagulants are used (see chapter on Anticoagulants). These include heparin, which is usually used in a hospital setting, as well as the oral drug, Coumadin (warfarin) and its derivatives.

drugs for preventing and treating arteriosclerosis

Finally, one of the major causes of cardiovascular problems comes from the formation of arteriosclerotic plaques in the arterial blood vessels. These plaques, made of fatty materials including cholesterol, can block the flow of blood to various tissues, such as the heart (eventually causing angina pectoris and coronary occlusion) or the brain (where blockage can cause a stroke). The actual mechanism of arteriosclerosis and the specific ways of preventing this plaque formation are not known. However, it is thought that a lower saturated fat and cholesterol intake may help prevent further plaque formation. Currently some drugs are used which are possibly effective in preventing arteriosclerosis in different ways and in different types of persons. These drugs, include Atromid and nicotinic acid (see Drugs for Arteriosclerosis). A further group of drugs is prescribed to increase circulation in areas already affected by arteriosclerosis. These include the drugs Hydergine, Pavabid and Vasodilan.

Drugs for high blood pressure

High blood pressure is one of the most common health problems in modern society, and many drugs are used to treat it. High blood pressure, also called hypertension, occurs when the pressure in the arterial blood vessels increases. The heart and blood vessels can be seen as a closed tubing system with a pump. The pressure in the system relates to how forcefully the pump works and the size and strength of the tubes, especially the arteries.

what is blood pressure?

The normal blood pressure in human arteries is a ratio usually less than 140/90 millimeters of mercury. (Mercury pressure is an arbitrary scale.) The upper figure, 140 in the example, is called the *systolic* pressure and measures the force of the heart, as well as indirectly the openness and strength of the arteries. The lower pressure, 90, is called the *diastolic* pressure and is the pressure when the heart relaxes (in diastole), and only the stiffness of the walls and the size of the arteries determine the pressure. Since the heart beats about 72 times per minute, in a person with a blood pressure of 140/90 there is a pressure of 140 in the system 72 times a minute as the heart beats, and a pressure of 90 between each beat.

high blood pressure

Hypertension occurs either when the heart contracts with more force and or when the arteries become smaller in diameter, usually due to constriction of the artery muscle walls. It can also occur when there is more fluid (or blood volume) in the system. A pressure of more than 140/90 in persons below the age of 60 and 160/90–95 in older persons (when taken on more than one occasion) is usually considered evidence of hypertension. The higher the pressure, the greater the problem. The reason why high blood pressure is harmful is that over periods of months to years this "pounding" type of pressure eventually damages small arteries and the organs that they supply, especially the brain and kidney. Also, of course, if affects the heart, since it has to pump against a higher pressure and do more work. Like any mechanical system that must work hard, it will eventually wear out. People with hypertension also have a higher incidence of other diseases and so its control can be seen as a form of preventive medicine.

One of the major determinants of blood pressure is the degree of contraction in the arterial blood vessels. This is controlled by many regulating substances in the body, as well as the nervous system. For example, blood pressure can rise due to an increase of activity in the sympathetic nervous system, which releases a substance called norepinephrine or noradrenaline (similar to adrenaline). This substance causes the arteries to constrict more tightly thus increasing the necessary force of heart contraction. Under stress, which may sometimes relate to periods of increased blood pressure, this system (also called the "fight or flight" nervous system because it prepares the body for these activities) is also activated. When this occurs, many people are aware of the heart "pounding," though they normally cannot feel the increased blood pressure. Many types of medicine, especially those used as general stimulants or appetite suppressants (such as amphetamines), or decongestants (such as Neosynephrine nasal sprays), or drugs used to treat asthma or allergies (such as epinephrine) have very similar effects on the arteries and can cause or aggravate high blood pressure. They can also interact with drugs used to treat high blood pressure.

All of the drugs used to treat high blood pressure act to block one or more of the causes of the increased blood pressure. Thus, they can either:

– decrease the volume in the closed system and/or

– block the sympathetic nervous system or one of the substances causing blood vessel constriction and/or

– dilate the arteries.

diuretics reduce fluid volume

The majority of antihypertensive drugs can be classified into three general categories. The first category is the diuretic drugs, which are usually the first drugs to be prescribed, and also represent the mainstay of therapy in many cases because they actually enhance the effect and benefit of other drugs. Prominent examples of diuretics include Hydrodiuril (hydrochlorothiazide) and Lasix (furosemide). Diuretics act to decrease the volume in the system by causing loss of excess water (often manifested as swelling of the feet, or edema) and salt. They also dilate, or enlarge, the blood vessels to some extent. By virtue of these two effects they are widely used alone to treat mild cases of raised blood pressure and in combination with other drugs in more severe cases. They are discussed and detailed in another section (see Diuretics).

nerve blockers

The second general category of drugs used in treating high blood pressure are called sympathetic blocking drugs. Reserpine, Aldomet and Ismelin are included in this category. Since the sympathetic nervous system can raise blood pressure by increasing the forcefulness of the heart contraction and forcing constriction of blood vessels, these drugs usually act on both to decrease slightly the heart's contracting force and rate, and to dilate blood vessels. The sympathetic nervous system originates in the brain and affects many other functions as well, such as bowel and bladder function and sexual response. This fact explains many of the side effects sometimes seen with these drugs that block the system, such as drowsiness, depression, change in sleep or dreaming patterns, diarrhea and change in sexual appetite. Since there is considerable variability in this system from person to person, dosage and side effects also vary widely.

blood vessel relaxers

The third category of drugs is the vasodilators, or blood vessel relaxing agents. They act only on the blood vessels to relax the walls and thus decrease pressure in the system. Apresoline (hydralazine) is the only drug in this category for oral prescription available in the U.S. at this time, although other vasodilators are used in emergency treatment of high blood pressure. This is a very effective way to lower blood pressure. but is dependent on the physical position of the person and is associated with some severe side effects after long-term use. Thus if a person stands suddenly, much of the blood will go into the lower part of the body, cutting the supply of blood going to the head, and the person may feel dizzy or faint. This is called postural hypotension, or low blood pressure due to change in position. After a few moments, the leg vessels and heart help readjust the circulation to bring the blood pressure back to normal. One type of readjustment is for the heart to beat rapidly and harder to increase the blood pressure, which can be a bothersome side effect. It can be blocked by sympathetic blocking drugs, so these are often given with vasodilators. Postural hypotension can also recur with some sympathetic blocking drugs; it is usually prevented by instructions to slowly change body position. This effect explains why a person with high blood pressure may get headaches when lying flat and why many doctors use positional changes in blood pressure to assess the effect of certain drugs.

combination drugs

Frequently high blood pressure is treated by a combination of diuretic, sympathetic blocker, and vasodilator. One of the major problems in drug therapy for hypertension is the need for a number of drugs, each of which must be taken several times a day. A person who started off with no symptoms may suffer from so many bothersome side effects that he feels worse then before. Accordingly, many persons fail to take their medication regularly and continue to have hypertension, which eventually may lead to stroke, kidney or heart failure.

One approach to this multiple drug problem has been the production of combination drugs for hypertension, so that one tablet contains drugs from two or all three categories (as for example, Aldoril and Aldactazide). Unfortunately, the establishment of an effective antihypertensive regimen often takes considerable adjustment to an individual drug, so use of combinations in initiating or changing therapy complicates this effort. Once a regimen is established, however, the combination preparations may be useful, as their convenience may outweigh their higher cost.

Another approach is to find drugs that act for a long time and that need only be taken once or twice daily. In some cases this is possible, especially in the treatment of mild hypertension. Unfortunately, in many cases drugs which are most effective and have the fewest side effects must be taken more frequently.

Listed below are some of the commonly prescribed drugs for high blood pressure. Those with an asterisk are individually described in Part III.

Aldactazide*	Dyrenium	Lasix*
Aldactone*	Enduron*	Regroton*
Aldomet*	Esidrex*	Renese-R
Aldoril*	hydrochlorothiazide*	reserpine
Apresoline*	Hydrodiuril*	Salutensin*
Catapres*	Hydropres*	Ser-ap-es*
Diupres*	Hygroton*	Serpasil
Diuril*	Inderal*	
Dyazide*	Ismelin*	

Diuretics ("water pills")

multipurpose "water pills"

Diuretic drugs are often referred to as "water pills" because they promote the loss of water, and salt, through the kidney into the urine. Common diuretic drugs include Hydrodiuril, hydrochlorothiazide, Lasix, Hygroton,

Dyazide, and Aldactazide. Diuretics are the mainstay in treatment of two very common disorders: high blood pressure and heart failure. They are also used to treat edema (swelling, usually of the feet and legs, but sometimes also of the hands, face or abdomen), kidney disease and liver disease (cirrhosis).

Diuretics have two related effects. The primary therapeutic effect of causing loss of water can prevent overloading the heart and blood vessels in high blood pressure and heart failure. Secondly, diuretics cause loss of salt (sodium chloride – the same as table salt). In many illnesses the kidney tends to retain salt and water in the body: diuretics act on the kidney to block this effect. Certain diuretics (Lasix, hydrochlorothiazide, Hydrodiuril) also cause loss of the essential salt, or mineral, potassium chloride, which must be replaced either through the diet, or by medicine supplement. Other diuretics, such as Dyazide, Aldactazide, Aldactone and Dyrenium, do not cause loss of potassium and are called potassium-retaining diuretics. Although potassium is not then required, these are not always considered drugs of choice because of other effects on the body's salt balance.

thiazide-type diuretics

Diuretics are commonly classified as thiazide type, potent diuretics, or potassium-retaining diuretics. Thiazide-type diuretics are so-called after their chemical class, which relates them to the sulfa drugs and the oral antidiabetic drugs. They are the most commonly used diuretics. Hydrochlorothiazide (Hydrodiuril, Esidrix) and the longer acting Hygroton are the most frequently prescribed. Hydrochlorothiazide is also included in many combination diuretics such as Dyazide and Aldactazide, and in combination antihypertensive drugs. Other thiazide-type diuretics are almost identical in their effects and side effects to hydrochlorothiazide, although some are longer acting. They include: Diuril, Enduron, Naturetin, Naqua, Oretic, Zaroxolyn, and Renese. Major side-effects of thiazide-type diuretics include a tendency to increase the blood sugar in people predisposed to diabetes, and to increase the uric acid content in blood, which can produce gout. They can all cause, in some persons, an excessive loss of water, potassium or sodium chloride. Thus, long-term therapy with any of these drugs usually requires occasional checks of blood values for sugar, uric acid and potassium. Occasionally, they can cause rashes or muscle cramps. If a true allergic reaction occurs against one member of this group, it may carry over to others, as well as to sulfa drugs.

The potent diuretics include Lasix (furosemide) and Edecrin (ethacrynic acid). Although Lasix is sometimes used in routine treatment of high blood pressure or heart failure, the potent diuretics are usually reserved for treatment of severe edema, as they can cause a loss of considerably more water and salt than the thiazide-type diuretics. The potent diuretics show many of the side effects of the thiazides, but they can also, rarely, lead to hearing problems, particularly if used with other drugs affecting the hearing nerves such as streptomycin or gentamicin.

The potassium-retaining diuretics, Dyrenium and Aldactone, are similar to thiazides but weaker. Because they don't cause potassium loss – eliminating the need to take extra potassium – they are often combined with a stronger thiazide diuretic as in Aldactazide (Aldactone plus hydrochlorothiazide) and Dyazide (Dyrenium plus hydrochlorothiazide). Although sometimes useful, they can be associated with some loss of kidney function and retention of too much potassium. Because of this Aldactazide has been found to have one of the highest incidences of side effects of all drugs used in hospitals. Such combination drugs are also usually more costly than hydrocholorthiazide.

A fourth kind of diuretic, Diamox, is essentially reserved for use in glaucoma therapy, partly because resistance to its effect develops rapidly and because it isn't particularly strong. It is useful in the treatment of glaucoma to reduce the water pressure in the eye, but it should only be taken intermittently.

Listed below are some of the commonly prescribed diuretics and diuretic-containing combinations. Those with an asterisk are individually described in Part III.

Aldactazide*	Hydrodiuril*	Regroton*
Aldactone*	Hygroton*	Salutensin*
Diamox Oral*	Lasix*	Ser-ap-es*
Diuril*		Renese-R
Dyazide*	**diuretic-containing**	
Dyrenium	**combinations**	
Enduron*	Aldoril*	
Esidrix*	Diupres*	
hydrochlorothiazide*	Hydropres*	

Drugs for heart failure

a bad example of
medical
terminology?

Undoubtedly one of the most emotive descriptions of any disease is the term "heart failure." But quite simply, heart failure means that the heart is failing to do its job efficiently, not that it has failed completely. Heart failure occurs in association with most other heart diseases since any failure of the circulatory pump can cause many changes. Except when the pump fails suddenly in an acute coronary occlusion (or heart attack), the changes are small. Often inefficiency results when the heart muscle doesn't get enough oxygen due to a clogged coronary artery, which carries blood and oxygen to the heart itself. At other times, there is too much blood and plasma for the heart to pump, or too much arterial pressure for the heart to pump against. The heart can also pump ineffectively if it beats too rapidly or irregularly, as in an arrhythmia. The most common arrhythmia is atrial fibrillation, which often occurs in conjunction with heart failure.

When the heart pumps inefficiently, a signal goes to the kidneys to retain water in order to keep up the pressure in the circulatory system. This is a protective mechanism in some acute situations such as shock, but otherwise it has a bad effect on the overloaded heart pumping system. The heart cannot pump all of the extra fluid, which then tends to accumulate in the legs (peripheral edema) or in the lungs (pulmonary edema). Meanwhile, the heart beats more rapidly. In very severe cases, the heart simply cannot get enough blood or oxygen to certain tissues, and they tend to look purplish or bluish.

shortness of
breath at
exercise or rest

Reduced blood circulation helps to explain some of the other symptoms of heart failure, especially shortness of breath, which accompanies even light exercise since the heart cannot supply the body with enough oxygen. Even while at rest, or at night, the lungs can become congested with edematous fluid, causing breathlessness. Swelling of the feet and legs occurs, as does the sensation of the heart beating rapidly. All of these rather predictable symptoms can indicate a failing heart. However, they can also occur in other conditions, and diagnosis must be confirmed by such tests as electrocardiograms and chest Xrays.

Since one acute problem is the presence of excess fluid in the lungs and elsewhere in the body, initial treatment often involves diuretics such as hydrochlorothiazide (Hydrodiuril, Esidrix) and Lasix (furosemide) to reduce the load

43

on the heart (see Diuretics). Often this alone will relieve many of the symptoms, but the specific causes of heart failure must be treated. If the heart has been pumping ineffectively owing to a rapid irregular rhythm, then slowing it to a normal rate will ease the problem. Similarly, if the heart has been forced to pump against very high pressure in the arteries, as in severe high blood pressure, then reducing pressure will cut the load. Occasionally, in severe heart failure, blood pressure and work for the heart is decreased by dilating the blood vessels. A defective heart valve obviously affects the heart's ability to pump, so repair or replacement of the valve surgically can sometimes remarkably improve functioning.

digitalis – a drug past its bicentennial

Sometimes, however, treatment of the specific causes of heart failure are not sufficient and the heart must be directly treated to improve its performance. In 1775, an English physician, William Withering, found that a local countrywoman was very successful at treating a condition called dropsy, which is characterized by severe edema, likely due to severe heart failure. Her treatment consisted of an herbal tea from the foxglove plant. Dr. Withering made good use of a chance observation and was instrumental in introducing the foxglove component, digitalis leaf, to modern therapy as the primary drug for heart failure. Today, digitalis, or its purified derivatives, continue as the mainstays in heart failure therapy. Digitalis drugs can overcome heart failure by actually increasing the strength of the heart's contraction. In addition, they improve the heart rate if it is rapid and irregular, which occurs in the very common abnormal rhythm called atrial fibrillation. Many persons rely on these dual effects of the digitalis drugs (Lanoxin, digoxin, digitoxin) to prevent recurring heart failure. They are discussed further in Section III.

Listed below are some of the commonly prescribed drugs for heart failure. Those marked with an asterisk are individually described in Part III.

digitalis digoxin* Lanoxin*

Drugs for abnormal heart rhythms

conditions that change the rhythm

The heart's muscle fibers are connected to an elaborate "wiring" or conduction system, that transmits electrical signals indicating the need for the muscle fiber to contract.

These signals are normally sent about 72 times every minute. The conductive system starts at the top of the heart, runs through the middle (septum) and spreads out through the heart walls. If the heart is damaged, as in a heart attack, or stretched, as in heart failure, impulse conduction can be affected, and the signal rhythm changed. If the conductive system is blocked or damaged, heart conduction can slow, or a type of "short-circuiting" can take place whereby the signals bypass the organized conduction system and "fire" more rapidly – sometimes irregularly, sometimes not. When normal conduction becomes disrupted, the abnormal heart rate and/or rhythm is called an *arrhythmia*. The drugs used to treat this condition are called anti-arrhythmic drugs, and they come from a wide variety of unrelated classes.

symptoms and dangers

Arrhythmias can be a problem for several reasons, and usually require treatment. If the heart goes too slowly, as in certain blocks of the conducting system, the supply of blood to the brain and other organs is not sufficient and the person may have fainting spells. Although this kind of arrhythmia is occasionally treated with drugs, if it persists it often requires the surgical placement of an artificial pacemaker.

On the other hand, several problems can occur if the heart goes too rapidly and/or irregularly. If the heart goes rapidly for a few minutes, it's usually no problem, although it may cause dizziness. However, when fast-beating persists, the heart is working less efficiently, resulting in heart failure (see Drugs for Heart Failure). Certain rapid rhythms can progress to very dangerous conditions, even cardiac arrest or heart stoppage. Other arrhythmias may by not be as rapid, but can lead to dangerous rhythms – a common occurrence just after a heart attack when the heart muscle and conductive system may be damaged. The drugs most commonly used in treating arrythmias include quinidine, Pronestyl, lidocaine (Xylocaine) and Inderal (propranolol). All of these drugs act in differ different ways on the electrical conduction affecting the heart, making it less likely to "short-circuit" or to conduct extra beats causing irregular rhythm.

Listed below are some of the commonly prescribed drugs for abnormal heart rhythms. Those with an asterisk are individually described in Part III.

Inderal*   quinidine*   Dilantin*
Pronestyl*   Xylocaine

Drugs used to prevent or treat circulation problems

blockage of the arteries

Arteriosclerosis describes a condition in which fat, cholesterol, and calcium deposits build up in the walls of arterial blood vessels. Eventually, this can lead to obstruction of those blood vessels, cutting off vital blood and oxygen supply to tissues. If the affected arteries serve the heart, partial obstruction and a decreased blood supply can lead to angina pectoris. If total obstruction occurs, the person has a heart attack. Similar obstruction of arteries to the head can cause strokes, while obstruction of arteries to the leg can cause eventual gangrene and loss of a leg if not treated.

The build-up of these fat-filled plaques is believed to occur gradually over many years, and some evidence points to the process starting in the early 20s. The process generally proceeds unnoticed until a catastrophic event such as a heart attack or stroke signals the presence of this ailment.

There is much controversy about the factors that cause this insidious build-up. Studies have identified several factors seemingly associated with arteriosclerotic disease, especially its early appearance (almost everyone has a fair amount of arteriosclerosis by the age of 80). These factors, called risk factors, include elevated levels of such fat substances in the blood as cholesterol and triglycerides, the presence of diabetes, a history of heavy smoking, a history of high intake of animal fats in meat and milk products, a history of high blood pressure, and – although still controversial – a history of high sugar intake and certain types of personality characteristics. Furthermore, a family history of early death (before age 55) from heart attack or stroke, or a history of elevated cholesterol or fat levels increases the likelihood of earlier problems with arteriosclerosis.

The medical approach to arteriosclerosis has been both preventive and therapeutic. There are some indications that preventive approaches may be having an impact in certain groups where there is a decreasing incidence of arteriosclerotic disease. This reduction has been attributed to various factors, the most prominent being the lower animal fat and cholesterol diet advocated by many heart associations and cardiologists for years: in fact, the true reasons are not known.

preventive drug
therapy
disappointing

Preventive drug therapy has been aimed at decreasing the amount of substances (such as cholesterol) available to make up the plaques. These efforts have been rather unsuccessful, although a number of drugs do reduce some types of blood fats, or lipids. One of the most commonly used is Atromid-S (clofibrate). Other drugs that have been tried include nicotinic acid, a thyroid hormone-like substance, Choloxin, estrogens, and drugs which prevent the absorption of fat and cholesterol from the bowel such as Questran (cholestyramine). Since cholesterol and other blood fats are key cellular building blocks, many drugs act to alter them while affecting other basic processes, so their lack of specific fat-reduction isn't too surprising. However, these and other drugs continue to be studied for their usefulness early in life, or on special subgroups that seem especially at risk. In the meantime, evidence continues to suggest that careful dietary regulation at an early age may play a key role in prevention.

A second approach to arteriosclerosis has been the attempt to prevent plaque formation and further obstruction which comes from formation of small clot-like material on the plaques. One of the common contibutors to such a clot is a type of blood cell, the platelet. When several platelets stick to a plaque, they can increase the obstruction. A group of drugs being extensively tested for prevention of recurrent strokes and heart attacks are the "antiplatelet" drugs, such as aspirin and Persantin, which decrease the stickiness of platelets. The usefulness of these drugs remains to be proven, but the small doses that seem necessary suggest this may be a relatively safe approach to some arteriosclerotic problems. Some physicians also use the blood-thinner, Coumadin, although because of its many problems, it is usually reserved for active clotting situations.

surgical removal
and plastic
bypass

The other major approach to arteriosclerosis is resorted to once there has been angina pectoris, a heart attack, a warning stroke, or poor circulation in the legs. Commonly, if the arteriosclerotic plaques are in large blood vessels, they can be surgically removed, or bypassed with dacron artificial arteries or veins (although arteriosclerotic plaques tend to form on these as well). Drug therapy, on the other hand, is directed at opening the arteries to improve circulation. Nitroglycerin has long been used to dilate arteries in the heart and elsewhere. Other drugs prescribed for opening up arteries elsewhere, which are somewhat more controversial, include Pavabid, Cerespan, Persantin, cyclospasmol, Vasodilan, and Hydergine. All of these have some ability to dilate some blood vessels when they are tested in experimental animals, although a number appear to be active only when injected. Few studies, however, demonstrate that the drugs, taken orally, can have much effect in arteriosclerosis. Nonetheless, they are widely used, and fortunately most have relatively few side effects, although they are often expensive.

Listed below are some of the commonly prescribed drugs for preventing or treating circulation problems. Those with an asterisk are individually described in Part III.

Attromid-S*	Hydergine*	Pavabid*
Cyclospasmol*	nicotinic acid*	Vasodilan*

Drugs for angina pectoris

what is angina pectoris?

Angina pectoris is an ailment in which a person suffers chest pains, below the breastbone, which are due to temporary lack of adequate blood supply, and therefore of oxygen, to the heart muscle. The usual cause of this pain is partial obstruction of the blood vessels, the coronary arteries, going to the heart muscle. The obstruction is often due to fat-containing arteriosclerotic materials called plaques, but also results from spasm of the coronary arteries. Attacks of angina pectoris occur more often with exercise, when the heart needs more oxygen in order to pump harder. It can also occur at rest, when it is usually associated with stress. Angina attacks may persist for months or years before obstruction or heart attack occurs, but this is quite unpredictable and a person with angina pectoris should therefore be under the direct care of a physician.

drugs for angina pectoris

Traditional drugs used to treat angina pectoris help prevent the attacks in two ways: 1) by opening up or dilating the coronary arteries to the heart (as is thought to be the case for the drug nitroglycerin), and 2) by decreasing the work the heart must do, especially in exercise. The most commonly used drugs in treating angina pectoris belong to a family of medication related to nitroglycerin, which includes Isordil and Peritrate. Nitroglycerin is taken in tablet form under the tongue, or in a paste on the skin, while the other drugs are taken orally and have a longer action. They are believed to act by both opening up the arteries to the heart, allowing a larger blood supply, as well as easing the load on the heart by opening up other blood vessels in the body.

Another type of drug used to treat angina pectoris is characterized by Inderal (propranolol) which decreases the work the heart must do, and thus decreases the angina pectoris. It is usually taken on a regular basis, but once started, it can only be discontinued gradually. Inderal belongs to a group of drugs called betablockers because they block the effects of certain stimulations aimed at increasing the heart beat rate. Betablockers are gaining acceptance for many heart conditions, as well as for hypertension.

change in
lifestyle just as
effective?

Frequently a person with angina pectoris will be on a general program for heart disease, which includes change in diet, smoking and drinking habits and exercise, as well as medication. Often one drug, such as Inderal, or Isordil, is taken on a regular basis, with nitroglycerin carried for use in the event of an acute attack. Each program should be highly individualized and supervised and reviewed with the physician on a regular basis. Especially when the primary cause of the attacks is stress, it is difficult to judge if successful treatment results from medication or the change in physical habits.

Listed below are some of the commonly prescribed drugs for angina pectoris. Those with an asterisk are individually described in Part III.

Inderal*   Nitrobid*   Sorbitrate*
Isordil*   nitroglycerine*

Anticoagulants ("Blood thinners")

There are three major types of drugs used to alter the body's blood clotting mechanism; heparin, which is only given by injection; coumarin-type drugs; and a third group called antiplatelet drugs, which includes aspirin. These drugs all act to prolong the time it takes blood to coagulate or clot and thus they prevent clot formation and are called *anticoagulants*. None of these drugs, however, actually dissolve clots which are already formed.

effects of blood clots

Prolonging the coagulation or clotting process may reduce the possibility of harmful clots forming and blocking the flow of blood in an artery, a vein, or the heart itself. The formation of such clots is called *thrombosis*, and the formation of a clot in an artery to the heart (a coronary artery) can cause a coronary thrombosis (a heart attack or myocardial infarction). A clot in the leg can also form in association with inflammation which is called *thrombophlebitis*. The clots that have formed on the inner surface of an artery or vein or in the heart may sometimes break loose and are carried by the blood flow to smaller blood vessels where they become wedged or trapped. This sequence is known as an *embolism*. For example, a clot from thrombophlebitis in the leg can break loose and travel to the lung and cause a pulmonary (lung) embolus, or blood clot in the lung.

Both thrombosis and or embolism are capable of decreasing the normal circulation of blood throughout the body, and if certain parts of the body are not receiving this vital supply of blood, those areas will become damaged and cease to function. In the case of a pulmonary embolus, the result is a damaged part of the lung. Reducing the possibility of obstruction or blockage of blood vessels by thrombosis or embolism with anticoagulants is believed to help reduce the likelihood of these life-threatening developments.

In the most common situation, when anticoagulants are used to prevent the progression of clots in the leg, or clots moving to the lung, a person is usually hospitalized and placed on the drug heparin which is given into the vein or by injection. After several days, the oral anticoagulant is started.

laboratory controls necessary

When anticoagulants are taken there needs to be very close medical supervision and doses must be highly individualized and adjusted during therapy. The effectiveness of anticoagulants varies from individual to individual, and even from time to time in the same person. Laboratory blood tests measuring the time it takes for the blood to clot before and during the administration of anticoagulants are used to determine the amount of drug the person must take to produce adequate results without risking complications. These laboratory tests are extremely important and must be done on a regular basis as long as the drug is taken.

complications

The most common complication of anticoagulation

therapy is bleeding, but this can usually be rapidly treated if a physician is notified immediately following minor bleeding. The common signs of bleeding are:

–red or dark brown urine, or less commonly, excessive menstrual bleeding.

–red or black bowel movements.

–uncontrollable bleeding of any kind (from shaving cuts, bloody nose or gums).

–unusually severe prolonged stomachache, headache or backache.

–sudden appearance of black-and-blue marks on the body.

interactions possible

Many drugs taken for completely unrelated conditions can greatly increase or decrease the degree of oral anticoagulant effects. Physicians and pharmacists are aware of these interactions but must be consulted beforehand and advised whenever *any* change in any drug regimen is planned. This includes any over-the-counter preparation and when prescription drugs are started, discontinued or changed in any way. It must also be remembered that certain foods in quantity, including green leafy vegetables such as spinach, cabbage and cauliflower, or multivitamin preparations containing vitamin K, affect anticoagulent therapy. Vitamin K can counteract the effect of the anticoagulant and this can encourage clotting. Therefore, major changes in eating habits, especially with the above foods and multivitamin preparations, should be discussed in advance with your physician.

The physician prescribing the oral anticoagulant should also be notified immediately if any other illness or injury occurs or if pregnancy is confirmed, or even suspected. Any physician, dentist or other health professional giving treatment to a person taking oral anticoagulants should be told of this fact. If long-term therapy is planned, the person should carry a card and or wear identification indicating that he is taking the drug.

The ability of aspirin and related drugs to prevent clotting, especially the type associated with strokes and heart attacks, by affecting one element of the blood, called platelets, has recently received attention and these drugs are currently being tested for therapeutic value. The effect on clotting is much less marked than the Coumadin type of drugs, so the hazards noted above generally do not apply. The use of aspirin as well as another drug, Persantin, in this way is still at the very early stage. When used, in low doses, they appear to be relatively safe, but whether they can help prevent strokes, heart attacks or other types of arteriosclerotic clotting remains to be seen.

Listed below are some of the commonly prescribed anticoagulants. Those with an asterisk are individually described in Part III.

aspirin*   heparin   Persantin
Coumadin*

Drugs for gastrointestinal disorders

the digestive
system

The digestive system begins at the mouth, teeth and salivary glands, and ends at the anorectal area. It is such a dynamic changing system, and its function of extracting vital nutrients and eliminating waste is so complex that it is not surprisingly a common site for problems, both major and minor.

Few persons can go through life without suffering some symptoms of nausea, vomiting, constipation or diarrhea. Consequently, there are an astounding number of preparations available by prescription or over-the-counter to relieve such symptoms. Frequently, the ailments associated with these symptoms are benign and self-limiting; sometimes they signal more serious problems such as ulcers, colitis and even cancer. Most drugs used for gastrointestinal complaints simply attempt to relieve the symptoms, with variable degrees of success; they can seldom affect the underlying cause, especially if it is serious or chronic. Sometimes dysfunction of the digestive, or gastrointestinal (G.I.) tract may be a reaction to stress, so that a queasy stomach or episodes of diarrhea may be common symptoms of anxiety. Nonetheless, any of the gastrointestinal symptoms, if recurrent, usually require medical evaluation to rule out serious causes. Many preparations used or prescribed for G.I. troubles act to relax the digestive tract muscles – the antispasmodic and antidiarrheal drugs. Many others aim to alter the actual contents of the G.I. tract: antacids, Maalox, Mylanta or Gelusil neutralize stomach acids; laxatives and some antidiarrheals, such as Kaopectate, change the bulk and content of the intestines, and help normalize its function. Few of these drugs are for long-term use since benign conditions often disappear after changes in the diet or relief of stress. Specific types of diseases and the drugs used for problems of the digestive tract are discussed in the next three sections.

Drugs for nausea, stomach upset and ulcers

causes of
stomach upset

Nausea, the sensation of stomach upset, and vomiting, can be due to a variety of causes. If these can be identified, they can be treated or prevented by relatively specific measures. Nausea can be due to a wide variety of problems, some as general as "gastrointestinal flu." Frequently a sensation of nausea or stomach upset can be due to irritation of the stomach lining because of an ulcer, or when a strong, irritating medicine is taken, for example, liquid potassium, high doses of theophylline (a drug for asthma), or aspirin. In these cases, direct treatment of the ulcer with antacids (see below) or preventing the irritation by diluting the medication with food or water may help avoid the symptoms.

Another occasional local cause of nausea or stomach distress may be over-distension or overfilling of the stomach with food or, not uncommonly, air that has been swallowed. Once considered, this seldom calls for drugs.

spasm of the
stomach and
antispasmodic
drugs

Vague stomach upset or vomiting is sometimes due to increased contraction of the muscle of the stomach, which can often give a sensation of a "knot in the stomach," hunger pangs, or nausea. This can, of course, be due to an ulcer or other local irritation, but often is associated with increased stomach contractions linked to stress. Although the exact mechanism is not known, these symptoms can often be relieved by antacids or by antispasmodic drugs such as Pro-Banthine, tincture of belladonna, or atropine. These drugs either act directly on the stomach or on the nerve to the stomach to decrease and slow contractions of the stomach and bowel, and may reduce secretions. Because these, as well as some symptoms of ulcer, are frequently associated with stress reactions, there are a number of antispasmodic drugs which are combined with tranquilizers, such as phenobarbital in Donnatal and Librium in Librax. Although extremely widely used, there is considerable question about these fixed combinations directed at two relatively *different* problems which need individual attention and dosing.

intolerance of
foods

Many persons become nauseated after eating certain foods. People with a tendency to have gallbladder disease may become nauseated after eating fatty foods, rich sauces or butter, or sometimes corn and cabbage. Others experience symptoms of intolerance and upset to a wide range of foods, such as spicy foods, coffee or dairy products. Although prevention is the key factor in this type of nausea, antacids will often, but by no means always, help.

nausea-
vomiting centers
in the brain

Frequently nausea and vomiting are due to irritation of four separate areas in the brain, including the vomiting center, an area called the chemoreceptor trigger zone and the vestibular apparatus in the inner ear, which is often affected in motion sickness or Meniere's syndrome. A number of drugs, such as codeine, morphine and certain anticancer drugs, directly affect these brain centers to cause vomiting. Fortunately, there are also a number of drugs that will stop or prevent nausea and vomiting due to these causes. Some of the most effective drugs for motion sickness are the various antihistamines (see Antihistamines) which act on the vestibular area. These include meclizine (Antivert, Bonine), Dramamine, Benadryl and hydroxyzine (Atarax, Vistaril). Nausea and vomiting due to stimulation of the other areas in the brain are sometimes helped by the antihistamines, but are also prevented with major tranquilizers such as Thorazine, Compazine or Phenergan, which are very effective, although these latter drugs in general have more potential side effects. An antispasmodic drug, scopolamine, is effective against most types of central vomiting. Tigan, is also used, but not for nausea due to inner ear or labyrinth irritation. In some cases, simple sedation with various tranquilizers is effective, but this is not usually appropriate and can be a problem if nausea and vomiting continue in a state of heavy sedation because it can cause aspiration – the breathing of vomitus into the lungs, which can cause severe pneumonia.

peptic ulcer and
its treatment

A peptic ulcer is a common, specific cause of stomach upset, and occasionally of pain, nausea and vomiting. An ulcer is essentially a breakdown in the mucus covered lining of the stomach, or the duodenum, which connects the stomach to the intestine. This breakdown of the tissue, which can be the size of a dime or much larger, can cause pain, spasm and bleeding. Ulcers can be very serious as heavy bleeding usually requires hospitalization and sometimes surgery. For this reason, early treatment at the first sign of an ulcer is essential.

The proper treatment of ulcers has long been a subject of debate in medical therapy, but at present it is felt that regular antacid therapy is of greater importance than a rigid diet in most cases. Although authorities still differ overall, most agree that coffee, alcohol and large amounts of spicy foods are not helpful.

The stomach is essentially a "bag" of hydrochloric acid in which food begins to be broken down by the strong acid and by an enzyme, pepsin, produced in the stomach. Any ulcer in this environment will be aggravated by the acid and enzyme; therefore, the primary goal in therapy is to neutralize the acid as continuously as possible with antacids. If an antacid is given and the stomach empties slowly, acid will be neutralized longer, which may justify the addition of the antispasmodic drugs, such as Pro-Banthine.

antacids

Several other aids can help achieve this goal of prolonged neutralization of acid in the stomach. First, liquid antacids are almost always more effective than tablets or chewed antacids. Second, especially in the presence of an acute ulcer, antacids may be needed very frequently (up to every 30 to 60 minutes) to prevent pain, and are usually needed at least every 2–3 hours. Third, antacids have a more prolonged effect when taken after food (food also neutralizes the stomach for a while) so it is useful to take antacid about an hour after meals, as well as every 2–3 hours thereafter. Fourth, acid secretions may increase at night, so a double dose of antacid and sometimes an antispasmodic drug at bedtime is often recommended.

other uses of antacids

Antacids come in a wide variety of compositions, tastes, and price. Most antacids contain one or more of the following salts: magnesium, calcium or aluminum. Because magnesium salts usually cause diarrhea when taken alone (for example, Milk of Magnesia is an antacid, but is more commonly used as a laxative!), and calcium and aluminum salts cause constipation on their own, the majority of antacids are made up as mixtures to avoid both side effects. Often, however, this is not the case and some experimenting with several antacids may be necessary to prevent constipation. Sodium bicarbonate is an effective antacid but cannot be used on a regular basis because it is absorbed and could cause problems with retention of the salt and alkali.

There is some argument about using the antacid calcium

carbonate (Dicarbosil and Titralac), because although very effective in neutralizing acid, once the effect wears off, there is increased acid secretion. If taken regularly, this isn't a problem. Sometimes, calcium can be absorbed, but this rarely causes difficulties except when a person drinks large quantities of milk over a long period (which can deposit calcium around bones) or takes diuretics such as hydrochlorothiazide (Esidrix or HydroDiuril) which can increase the level of calcium in the blood.

Because part of their function is to protect the stomach lining and neutralize acids, many antacids prevent absorption of drugs, so that taking drugs with antacids should be avoided, and any medication should be taken on an empty stomach between antacid use.

Antacids are also used, as noted above, for simple gastric upset after a heavy or spicy dinner, or too much alcohol (heartburn, acid indigestion) and more often than not serve to relieve the symptoms. In conditions of hiatus hernia (where the stomach extends slightly above the diaphragm), and of acid reflux, stomach acids often back up into the esophagus and can cause belching and heartburn, especially at night. These symptoms are often completely relieved by the use of antacids after the evening meal and at bedtime, along with the precaution of not reclining until at least three hours after eating, and raising the head of the bed. In kidney failure certain antacids containing aluminum, such as Basajel and Amphojel, are used to prevent accumulation of phosphorus, since they bind it in the intestine.

antispasmodics

Antispasmodic drugs, such as tincture of belladonna or Pro-Banthine, are also useful in ulcer therapy to decrease spasm of the stomach, and also to partially block the hypersecretion of acid and pepsin. Antispasmodic drugs are likewise used in similar disorders where increased stomach or bowel spasm is a problem – an exception being hiatus hernia and acid reflux, which antispasmodics may make worse.

There are a large number of antispasmodic drugs available, most of them acting as anticholinergic drugs to block signals to the vagus nerve, which increases acid secretion and contraction of the stomach. These antispasmodic, anticholinergic drugs act elsewhere in the body, so along with effects on the stomach they may cause dryness in the mouth, blurring of vision, and difficulty with urination at higher doses. Since a person can seldom feel effects of medication on the stomach, the presence of a dry mouth is usually a good indication that the drug is working, and is used as such. Usually these drugs are taken before meals and or at bedtime. The bedtime dose may be most useful as it can help retain the antacid taken at night in the stomach (which it slows down) and decreases the need for antacids in the middle of the night. Antispasmodic drugs may cause retention of urine in men with prostate trouble, so they are used with caution, if at all, in elderly men. They can also counteract the drugs used in glaucoma, so are likewise used cautiously in that condition.

Listed below are some of the commonly prescribed drugs for nausea, stomach upset and ulcers. Those with an asterisk are individually described in Part III.

Amphogel	Combid*	Mylanta
Antivert*	Compazine*	Pro-Banthine*
Basalgel	Donnatal*	Tigan*
Bentyl*	Gelusil	TUMS
Bentyll Phenobarbital*	Librax*	
Bendectin*	Maalox	

Drugs for constipation

the constipation fixation

Constipation, commonly defined as difficult, infrequent evacuation of the bowel, has been a preoccupation of advanced societies for years. For a long time, daily evacuation of the bowels was believed to prevent virtually all disease, but we can now be absolutely certain that good health does not require regular bowel movements at fixed times. Normal bowel function can range from three bowel movements a day to three a week or even less.

The last few decades have seen a dramatic decrease in the routine use of cathartics by the medical profession, but self-prescribed laxatives still enjoy widespread use by the general public, and a large majority still remain "bowel conscious." This is confirmed by the availability of more than 700 different laxative products, on which over $400 million is spent annually. General misconceptions about normal bowel function and extensive advertising by pharmaceutical manufacturers contribute to the overuse, misuse and abuse of self-prescribed laxatives.

Simple constipation most frequently results from the wrong sort of diet, insufficient intake of liquids, sometimes a change in habits because of travel, and perhaps insufficient exercise. Laxatives are rarely indicated for relief of simple constipation: relief can be achieved by changing to a better quality diet which includes foods with a higher fiber content, adequate liquid intake, and prompt response to the urge to evacuate the bowels.

Constipation can have a relatively sudden onset because the condition may result from a pre-existing disease, such as hypothroidism (decreased thyroid function), cancer of the colon, and some types of depression. Constipation may also be caused by many drugs, including certain antacids, narcotic analgesics (such as codeine), anticholinergics, antispasmodics, some tranquilizers and antidepressants, and preparations containing iron.

The terms laxative, cathartic, and purgative are often confused: all three describe agents that act to bring about a bowel movement, but these agents differ in degree of action. A cathartic is slightly more active than a purgative, but the two terms are relatively interchangeable since both types of agent rapidly produce bowel evacuation and a definite change in stool consistency, often watery feces. These actions are less pronounced in the case of a laxative, although a suffficiently large dose of laxative can produce a cathartic effect.

Laxatives can be classified into several groups:
– Bulk forming laxatives
– Stimulant laxatives
– Lubricants (mineral oil)
– Stool softeners.

The various, frequently prescribed laxative products are discussed here in the appropriate category, although some products contain more than one type of active ingredient.

bulk forming laxatives

Bulk forming laxatives promote bowel evacuation (bowel movement) by increasing the mass of the stool and by softening the stool through their ability to attract and hold water within it. The increased bulk of the stool usually increases the frequency of bowel movements. These laxatives are generally not absorbed from the gut and do not appear to have any influence on the absorption of nutrients from food. They are considered the safest laxatives. A bulk forming laxative may take from one to three days to have an effect, so that to maintain a consistent result, they should be taken three or more times a week.

The major precaution to observe when taking any bulk

forming laxative is to take adequate fluid with each dose (at lease eight fluid ounces of water) to ensure that the laxative does not form a hard, obstructing lump in the intestinal tract.

Bulk forming laxatives come from two main sources. The least costly source is crude dietary fiber, including bran, whole fruits, leafy vegetables, raw carrots and wholegrain breads. Most others are made from semisynthetic cellulose derivatives, such as psyllium (obtained from Plantago seed), and methylcellulose.

Common bulk forming products include Dialose, Effersyllium, Hydrocil, Metamucil, and Serutan. All work in a similar way: the major differences relate to cost and personal preference.

stimulant
laxatives
Stimulant laxatives increase the wavelike (peristaltic) contractions of the intestinal musculature which pushes the bowel content along in the direction of the wave. These drugs were so-named because they were believed to stimulate the nerves of the gut and to irritate the lining of the intestine as well as having a direct effect on the muscles. But stimulant laxatives also cause more fluid to enter the intestine – which in itself will stimulate increased peristalsis. Their exact mechanism of action in causing evacuation of the bowel, is, therefore, not completely determined.

The potency of different stimulant laxative products varies greatly according to the response of the individual. A bowel movement usually occurs after about six hours. Stimulant laxatives should be used only occasionally and never more than daily for one week to relieve simple constipation. If stimulant laxatives are used for a long period, normal bowel function can be lost and the individual may become dependent on the drug for bowel evacuation.

Noticeable side effects of these laxatives include intestinal cramps and burning, diarrhea, and depletion of body water (dehydration). Some stimulant laxatives are eliminated by the kidneys after absorption from the gut and can produce colored urine. In general terms, this group of laxatives is considered the least desirable because of the unpleasant side effects and the tendency to alter bowel function after extended use.

Bisacodyl (Dulcolax) is a stimulant laxative available only on prescription in either tablet or suppository form. The suppository induces a bowel movement approximately

15 minutes to an hour after insertion, while tablets usually produce an effect overnight – 6 to 12 hours after being taken. To avoid irritation of the stomach lining due to premature dissolving, Dulcolax tablets must be swallowed whole – not chewed – and should not be taken within an hour of taking antacids or milk.

Many stimulant laxative drugs are derivatives of a substance called anthraquinone, a family of natural ingredients including cascara sagrada (literally sacred bark from the buckthorn tree *Rhamnus purshiana*), senna (dried leaflets of the *Cassia* plant), and aloe (a leaf extract). Similar to these natural forms is a synthetic compound, danthron (Dorbane, Modane). Danthron tablets are available without prescription and must be swallowed whole in a similar way to Dulcolax. Common anthraquinone laxatives include Black Draught, Carter's Little Liver Pills, Cas-Evac, Fletcher's Castoria, and Senokot.

Phenolphthalein is another type of stimulant laxative compound and is a common ingredient of many products, including Ex-Lax, Feen-a-Mint, Phenocal and Veracolate.

saline laxatives

Saline laxatives, such as Milk of Magnesia, are chemical salts that hold water within the gut and so indirectly stimulate peristalsis. A bowel movement usually occurs within one or two hours with a sufficient dose of the laxative. Saline laxatives can be regarded as safe and effective only when used occasionally. Continuous use for more than a week may cause serious side effects mainly due to dehydration and/or loss of essential minerals.

The commonest saline laxatives are Milk of Magnesia (magnesium hydroxide suspension), Epsom Salts (magnesium sulfate), Fleet's Phospho-Soda (sodium phosphate), and Sal Hepatica (more than 50% sodium biphosphate). Citrate of magnesia (magnesium citrate) – often used to clear the bowel as a preliminary to Xray examination – should be stored in a refrigerator to slow down decomposition, but in general, these products are relatively stable and require no special storage.

Magnesium contained in saline laxatives can be absorbed into the blood and may produce undesirable effects. For example, in patients with kidney disease, the magnesium can build up to toxic levels in the body and cause depression of the central nervous system (sedation and confusion) and weakness of the skeletal muscles. These preparations should, therefore, be avoided by people with inadequate kidney function.

Sodium can be similarly absorbed, so that laxatives containing sodium chloride, such as Fleet's Phospho-Soda or Sal Hepatica, should be avoided by patients with any illness that requires salt restriction, including heart conditions, or any diseases with edema or high blood pressure.

Mineral oil is a colorless, tasteless mixture of liquids that has enjoyed popular use as a laxative. Whether mineral oil lubricates the intestinal tract is unknown, but the oil softens the stools and promotes their easier evacuation. Mineral oil preparations are non-irritating and only slightly absorbed. The usual dose is one or two tablespoons taken at bedtime on an empty stomach. With proper and careful use, mineral oil produces few side effects, but these laxative preparations should be strictly reserved for very occasional use.

Several problems can arise through the use of mineral oil. If taken with food in the stomach, a theoretical risk exists that the oil may impair the absorption of fat soluble nutrients including vitamins A,D,E, and K. A common annoyance, especially with excessive quantities, is oozing of the oil from the anorectum; anal irritation may also occur.

A significant problem can occur if mineral oil is given to someone lying on his back: the oil may be inhaled into the lungs and cause the serious condition of lipid (fat) pneumonia. Inhalation is most likely to occur in very young, debilitated, or elderly bedridden persons, and for these cases mineral oil is best avoided. Whenever mineral oil is used, all precautions should be taken to ensure that it is completely swallowed and is not likely to be regurgitated later (a good reason for not taking mineral oil late at night).

lubricants
(mineral oil)

Mineral oil is available in simple or emulsified forms, such as Agoral, Haley's M-O, and Kondremul. Emulsification reduces the size of the oil droplets and enhances penetration of the oil into the feces, but at the same time, intestinal absorption of the oil is increased. Emulsions are usually given as two daily doses, one on rising and one at bedtime, but never at mealtimes. All precautions mentioned also apply to mineral oil emulsions.

Mineral oil should not be given at the same time as stool softening laxatives, because absorption of the oil may be enhanced.

Stool softeners are the most recently developed laxatives. Their detergent action facilitates the penetration of intestinal fluids (primarily water) into the stool, which is softened and so more easily passed out of the bowel. The effects are apparent only one to three days after ingestion. For beneficial and consistent effects, stool softeners therefore need to be taken at least three times a week, although not for long, continuous periods. These laxatives should be used only occasionally for simple constipation and, in any event, no more than daily for one week.

At present, only occasional insignificant side effects have been attributed to stool softeners, but these drugs are believed to have some action on the lining of the intestine to enhance the secretion of water (which would aid the laxative effect) and affect the absorption of other compounds (as has been demonstrated with mineral oil). Stool softeners may well interact with other drugs and affect absorption of some nutrients.

stool softeners

Stool softeners are available in forms suitable for rectal or oral administration. The usual dose is 100 to 250 mg daily, but the dose should generally be the smallest possible that produces the desired effect.

The most frequently prescribed laxatives – dioctyl sodium sulfosuccinate, known by the brand names Colace, Doxinate, and Peri-Colace, or as D.S.S. – are stool softeners. Dioctyl sodium sulfosuccinate is the most popular stool softening drug and is marketed by numerous pharmaceutical companies in various strengths in capsule, solution and syrup forms. These preparations can also be bought under their generic name over the counter from pharmacies with a substantial saving in cost compared with the better known branded preparations of the same drug. For example, Colace and Doxinate are two of the most frequently advertised and prescribed brand name preparations of dioctyl sodium sulfosuccinate; they cost about seven times as much as the same drug bought generically.

a combination laxative

Peri-Colace is a combination product that contains 100 mg dioctyl sodium sulfosuccinate plus 30 mg of the anthraquinone stimulant laxative casanthranol (Peristim): the idea is to combine the stimulant and stool softening properties of the two ingredients. The undesirable feature of Peri-Colace, as with most other combinations, is that both ingredients are always present and must be taken together, even if one effect is not required.

The potential dangers of chronic abuse of stimulant laxatives have already been mentioned, and these apply equally strongly to casanthranol in this combination. In addition, Peri-Colace is one of the most expensive laxatives available. The rational approach is to use a stimulant or saline laxative as required, and to add dioctyl sodium sulfosuccinate only when really needed.

Drugs for diarrhea

Diarrhea can be defined as the passage of bowel movements with increased frequency and with increased water content. Normal bowel movements contain approximately 60 – 70% water, but in the case of diarrhea, they contain up to 80 – 95% water. When diarrhea occurs, there is usually an increased movement of the circular muscles of the bowel walls, which in wavelike contractions (peristalsis) "rushes" food and fluids through the gastrointestinal tract. This prevents their proper digestion and absorption into the body and accounts for the increased fluid and undigested food particles seen with diarrhea.

causes of diarrhea

Causes of diarrhea include bacterial and viral infections, parasite infestations, diseases of the intestine such as ulcerative colitis, and hormonal disturbances, to name just a few. Diarrhea is often accompanied by loss of appetite, abdominal cramps due to the contractions of the bowel and trapped gas, and nausea and vomiting, which is also usually due to the increased contraction of the muscles in the gastrointestinal tract. The increased contraction is often due to irritants or toxins from the bacteria. This is a common cause of the diarrhea seen with food poisoning, and in traveler's diarrhea. Sometimes, increased stress can also cause intermittent diarrhea. Certain foods commonly produce diarrhea in certain persons. For example, a large percentage of the adult population has no enzyme to digest milk products normally. This commonly can produce diarrhea which is relieved by avoiding milk products. Other foods, such as coffee (in excess), spicy or fatty foods may produce diarrhea. Diarrhea can also occur due to an irritant in the bowel – this can signal a serious ulcer, or even tumor, which is one of the reasons diarrhea should be evaluated if it persists for more than 2 to 3 days.

Another reason that persistent diarrhea requires medical attention is that it can cause significant loss of water and salt from the body and produce deydration. This is particularly true of infants and elderly persons. Diarrhea may also prevent absorption of certain drugs, such as oral contraceptives or anticonvulsants, so that loss of their effects can occur. The experience of diarrhea is quite uncomfortable, unsociable and often embarrassing, so that immediate symptomatic relief is often sought.

action of antidiarrheal drugs

Antidiarrheal products act to decrease diarrhea in two general ways. One type of product which includes drugs such as Kaopectate, acts to increase the bulk of the stool, and also possibly absorb some of the toxins contributing to the increased movement or irritability of the bowel. The other type of drug, such as Lomotil, tends to act directly on the bowel muscle and decreases contractions, thus slowing the movement of material through the gastrointestinal tract. These drugs all provide symptomatic relief and do not usually affect the cause of the diarrhea. They are most effective in the mildest forms of diarrhea.

Prolonged use of an antidiarrheal preparation without identification of the underlying cause may result in serious complications. For this reason, symptomatic relief of undiagnosed diarrhea for more than two days is not recommended and proper examination by a physician is then advisable. All of the products described below provide purely symptomatic relief, and should not be used more than two to three consecutive days without a physician's directions.

Listed below are some of the commonly prescribed drugs for diarrhea. Those with an asterisk are individually described in Part III.

Donnagel-PG*   Lomotil*   paregoric
Kaopectate*

Hormonal drugs

what is a hormone?

A hormone is commonly defined as a substance or chemical produced in the body by organs called endocrine glands, thus the name endocrinologists for medical specialists dealing with gland troubles. The endocrine glands include the thyroid, the parathyroid, the adrenal, the pancreas, the ovary and the testicle. The hormones produced by these glands, such as the thyroid hormone made by the thyroid gland, are released to the blood stream and travel to other organs and tissues to regulate or modify their function. Thus, the thyroid hormone regulates the speed of metabolism of most cells; insulin from the pancreas regulates the usage of sugar by the cells; estrogen from the ovary helps regulate the menstrual cycle.

the master
gland: the
pituitary

The amounts of hormones released from the gland are very carefully controlled, in most instances by the so-called master gland, the pituitary. This gland, located at the very center of the head, behind the nose and eyes, releases specific, special hormones (called tropic hormones) that go to the glands to signal how much of each hormone to release. Some of these tropic hormones are actually used as drugs or by clinicians as tests for gland function. An important example is ACTH, which stands for adrenocorticotropic hormone, meaning the hormone which stimulates the adrenal gland to release cortisone-like hormones.

The pituitary gland, in turn, gets its signals from a part of the brain, the hypothalamus, which monitors the hormones circulating in the blood. If the hormone level is low, signals (again in the form of a special type of hormone) go to the pituitary gland to cause release of tropic hormone to tell the gland to produce more of the deficient hormone. If a certain hormone level is high or if a hormone is used in high doses, as in a drug, the pituitary gland signals the gland to decrease the amount released. If this continues for long periods, the gland may become less active (atrophy) and may require weeks or months to recover if the need for hormone secretion is decreased. The general scheme thus comprises a full feedback cycle and allows for very careful regulation of hormone levels.

two uses of
hormones:
replacement and
as drugs

Hormones are given for two general purposes. First, they are used as replacement therapy to provide normal hormone levels when a gland has been removed (as when the thyroid is removed) or damaged by disease (as in diabetes, where the pancreas cannot produce enough insulin). In general, hormones are given in doses similar to those normally produced in the body and administered on the same time scheme as well, for example, the adrenal secretes cortisone in the morning, so it is usually given then. Replacement therapy is given to replace thyroid, adrenal, ovarian (female, estrogen and progesterone), testicular (male, androgen or testosterone) and pancreatic gland secretions. The parathyroid hormone is not usually given, but since it regulates calcium metabolism, calcium is prescribed instead. The most common hormone deficiencies are those of thyroid, insulin and female hormones; these are discussed further in the following essays. Deficiencies of other hormones are much less common and are not discussed here.

hormones as
drugs

The second type of hormone therapy involves use of the hormone in higher-than-usual doses (pharmacological doses), as a drug. Synthetic hormones resembling cortisone, such as prednisone, are most commonly used in this way. Many uses of estrogen, including oral contraceptives, also fall into this category (see Oral Contraceptives; Estrogens and Progestogens used in Hormone Therapy). This type of therapy does tend to interfere with normal gland function because of the feedback cycle described above; therefore the monitor in the brain registers high hormonal levels, and generates signals to the pituitary gland and to the primary glands to decrease their function. For example, the ovaries get smaller when oral contraceptives are taken. So when these hormones are stopped, it may take weeks or months for the ovaries to return to normal function.

Drugs for thyroid disorders

importance of
the thyroid

The thyroid is an endocrine gland located in the neck in front of the windpipe. Its primary function is to produce the thyroid hormone called thyroxin. Thyroxin is made from a simple amino acid and iodine, which is one reason why the proper amount of iodine in the diet is critical. Thyroid hormone circulates through the entire body and acts on most cells to regulate their metabolism – their turnover of oxygen and nutrients. In the fetus it may also affect the development of certain organs including the brain. Diseases of the thyroid may or may not cause changes in the amount of thyroid hormone produced.

treatment of an
overactive
thyroid gland

If an excess amount of thyroid hormone is produced, a person may feel continually warm, sweaty, shaky, and experience diarrhea, nervousness, palpitations and changes in the skin or hair. This is usually the result of increased function of the gland, which is often enlarged, and the most usual treatment is by radioactive iodine therapy or surgery. Occasionally certain drugs are used either prior to surgery or alone in an attempt to control the disease. If surgery is planned, iodine or iodide solution is sometimes used along with one of the anti-thyroid drugs, either propylthiouracil or Tapazole (methimazole). Occasionally, when the symptoms are very severe, the drugs propranolol (Inderal) or guanethidine (Ismelin) have been used for short periods of time to decrease the palpitations and nervousness.

treatment of an

The condition where there is under-secretion of thyroid

underactive
thyroid gland

hormone, either due to removal of the gland or decreased function, is called hypothyroidism. This condition, with lower amounts of thyroid hormone, can result in slowed metabolism, which can cause lethargy or tiredness, increased sensitivity to cold, constipation, and dullness or dryness of the skin or hair. When this is discovered, usually by measuring levels of thyroid hormone in the blood, thyroid is given as replacement therapy. If true deficiency is established, it is usually taken for life. For many years, the source of thyroid hormone was the dehydrated thyroid glands of cows or pigs, and thyroid pills were the primary drug used. Although the amount of thyroid hormone present was tested, the actual amount tended to vary from lot to lot. Thus, when the purified hormone, thyroxin (used in Synthroid) became available more recently, it quickly became the preferred form.

erroneous use of
thyroid in weight
reduction

Thyroid therapy has unfortunately found use in many programs for weight loss since the thyroid hormone increases metabolism and the rate of use of foodstuffs. In all cases except where true deficiency of hormone has been found by blood tests, the use of such therapy is inappropriate and can cause problems, especially if there is a risk of heart disease.

Listed below are some of the commonly prescribed drugs for thyroid disorders. Those with an asterisk are individually described in Part III.

Cytomel*   Synthroid*   thyroid*
Proloid*   Tapazole

Drugs for diabetes

what is diabetes
mellitus?

Diabetes mellitus is a complex disease associated with two major abnormalities. First, it is characterized by high blood sugar (hyperglycemia) and other change in use of foodstuffs due to either a lack of, or an inability to use the hormone insulin, which comes from the pancreas gland. Second, it is characterized by an abnormality of tiny blood vessels throughout the body, which over long periods of time produces abnormalities of many organs, such as the eyes, the kidneys and nerves.

two types of
diabetes:
insulin-dependent
and adult-onset

There are two very general types of diabetes which differ considerably in their severity, their treatment, and age of onset. "Classical" diabetes is associated with a partial or complete lack of insulin, usually starts (often abruptly) before age 30 or 40, and requires insulin therapy. For this reason it is often termed insulin-dependent diabetes. It is also called juvenile diabetes because it often starts in the teenage years. This type of diabetes is more likely to be associated with a very serious condition called ketoacidosis (usually requiring hospitalization) which may occur with stress, infection, or inadequate insulin therapy.

The other, much more common type of diabetes often termed maturity or adult-onset diabetes, is not necessarily due to an absolute lack of insulin, but rather a dysfunction of the pancreas in releasing insulin and or inability of the body to use the insulin properly. It is more often seen in persons over age 40 and more frequently in overweight persons. Only 10 – 20% of persons with this type of diabetes actually require insulin, and sometimes only when they become otherwise ill. Most people with this type of diabetes can be treated by diet and weight loss, although a few may need oral antidiabetic drugs as well. People suffering from this type of diabetes seldom "get out of control" with ketoacidosis and seldom require hospitalization for their diabetes except for late-stage complications such as foot ulcers and arteriosclerosis.

The treatment of diabetes has several goals – some are readily achieved, others are more difficult. The two major objectives are to allow the person to live a relatively normal life for a normal span with few complications. There is considerable controversy among experts in diabetes as to which goal is more important, since there is a potential conflict. Thus, "normalization" of activity and diet may or may not prolong life. Conversely, procedures aimed at "control" of diabetes, such as a very rigid diet, which are believed to prolong life and prevent complications, may interfere with what we think of as a normal life. Most regimens in fact address both goals and try to achieve a happy medium, but these factors require discussion with the physician.

specific therapy goals

More specific goals in treatment generally relate to those factors which cause problems and complications in diabetes. These include: (1) prevention of "spilling" excess sugar in the urine by use of diet and/or insulin and/or antidiabetic drugs; (2) prevention of infection by avoidance of exposure, adequate vaccination and special care with hygiene; (3) prevention of excess lowering of blood sugar (hypoglycemia) and (4) prevention of the arteriosclerosis and vascular changes associated with many of the longer-term problems, such as foot ulcers and arterial blockage.

preventing spillage of sugar

There is considerable argument over whether there should be close control of the amount of sugar in the blood or not, although most experts agree that continual spillage of sugar in the urine is not desirable. Some background will help: when food is eaten, the foodstuffs are converted in part to sugar and travel throughout the body to the cells, where the sugar provides energy. The sugars cannot easily enter the cell without the hormone insulin, which is released from the pancreas shortly after food is eaten. If there is not enough insulin, the sugar will stay in the blood and the level will be higher than normal for several hours after eating. If it becomes very high, it will spill over into the urine. Therefore, sugar in the urine usually indicates that the blood level is too high (though rarely this only means that the kidney is "leaky" and the urine will contain sugar while the blood sugar is normal). When sugar goes into the urine, a certain amount of body water must go out with it to dilute it. If the blood sugar stays high and sugar and water continue to go out in the urine, the person can lose too much water and become dehydrated. This can result in increased urination (due to the extra water loss) and also increased thirst. If this continues, a person's body metabolism changes in order to get energy from other foodstuffs and this can result in the beginnings of ketoacidosis – one of the most serious complications of diabetes. Therefore, it is usually agreed that the amount of sugar spilled in the urine should be kept to a minimum.

testing urine for sugar

Because of this agreement, most diabetics are taught to check their urine for sugar using tablets (Clinitest) or paper strips (Diastix or Tes-Tape). They are also sometimes asked to check for acetone, (an early sign of ketosis) with Ketostix, Acetest or Keto-Diastix. In persons with insulin-dependent diabetes, urine testing may be done frequently; it is usually checked less often in most adult-onset diabetics. The testing and the expected results should be thoroughly discussed and understood by the patient. Most physicians prefer the diabetic to keep a chart to monitor therapy, as this is the primary way in which correct doses of insulin or other drugs are established. Clinitest tablets can give a false positive result in the presence of certain drugs, such as high doses of vitamin C (more than one gram per day) or the antibiotic Keflex, so other tests, such as the Tes-Tape or Diastix must be used.

regulation of
blood sugar

It is not known how helpful it is to lower blood sugar that is higher than normal but not high enough to cause spillage into the urine. Attempts to regulate a diet, which is the mainstay of all diabetic therapy, will often alone prevent blood sugar from becoming excessively high, but in insulin-dependent diabetics, insulin is also required. If insulin is used to regulate the blood sugar very closely, there is often the danger of dropping the blood sugar too low and causing an insulin reaction (hypoglycemia). Most physicians prefer to regulate the diet, and use insulin or oral drugs in doses sufficient to prevent spilling large amounts of sugar into the urine (the majority of diabetics do occasionally spill sugar) without lowering the sugar so far as to cause frequent hypoglycemic attacks.

diet therapy

Because diabetes is a disease of the metabolism, which limits the flexibility of the body in handling various foodstuffs, the base of all therapy and prerequisite for either insulin or oral antidiabetic therapy is a well-rounded controlled diet. The specifics of diet therapy are discussed in many books on the subject and should be well understood by the person who has been diagnosed as diabetic. Suffice it to say that diabetic diets aim to maintain optimal body weight (which usually entails dieting for adult-onset diabetics who are frequently overweight) and at the same time provide the necessary carbohydrates, fat and protein while preventing hyperglycemia, ketoacidosis or hypoglycemia.

insulin therapy

Prior to the discovery of insulin in the 1920s, the outlook for persons with insulin-dependent diabetes was very bleak. Therefore, the discovery that this protein hormone could be extracted from the pancreas of pigs and cows for treatment was a great medical advance. There have been many refinements since and insulin is now available in several forms, primarily differentiated by onset and length of action. The short-acting "regular" insulin is commonly used when treatment is first started and to give control during stress or illness, usually in the hospital. For chronic or long-lasting therapy, such intermediate-acting forms of insulin as NPH or Lente, are used, which often require only one injection a day. Longer-acting insulins are used rather infrequently. Insulin is measured by units – a unit standing for a certain amount of a biological (blood sugar lowering) activity. Insulin is destroyed in the stomach, so it must always be given by injection, usually into the fatty (subcutaneous) tissue of the arms or legs. When insulin injections are first started, local itching and redness may be seen, but this usually disappears in a few weeks. A person is taught to rotate injection sites to prevent damage to the skin.

Insulins are now available in three concentrations: U-40, U-80 and the newer, more concentrated U-100 form. Because of some confusion over the various concentrations of insulin, it is usually being recommended that all diabetics convert to the standard form, U-100 insulin, which has specially measured syringes. In the future, this will help avoid errors or confusion associated with differing concentrations.

problems of insulin therapy

The use of insulin is associated with some problems, the primary one being establishing the best type of insulin (i.e. intermediate acting with or without "regular" insulin) as well as establishing the proper dose and schedule for use. With three meals a day, the blood sugar will rise three times a day, the height depending on how much is eaten and how much insulin is available. Frequently, a person is put on a dose of intermediate insulin, such as NPH, which is injected in the morning. It begins to act in two hours (on the blood sugar due to breakfast) and has its peak of action eight to ten hours later near the time of the evening meal. If a person eats no lunch, then the blood sugar may get so low that a hypoglycemic reaction (with symptoms of shakiness, dizziness, lightheadedness or sweating) may occur. This is always treated by taking some type of readily available sugar, (as in a sugar cube, orange juice or candy bar – the only instance where this high sugar food is appropriate in a diabetic diet). A diabetic on insulin should usually carry some source of readily available sugar for this purpose, as advised by his physician. In some cases, there is a need to give a shorter acting, regular insulin in the morning to cover the effects of breakfast and lunch. Occasionally, good control is only obtained when insulin is given twice daily. *This must always be determined individually*, usually using urine testing as a guide. The requirements of any individual tend to stabilize, but may change with diet, exercise and the presence of infection.

oral antidiabetic drugs

In the early 1960s, the introduction of a new group of drugs, some chemically related to sulfa drugs and thiazide diuretics, promised the potential of oral therapy for diabetics which would eliminate the need for insulin in many cases. Two general types of drugs were introduced: The *sulfonylurias* which include Orinase (tolbutamide),

Tolinase (tolazamide), Diabinese (chlorpropamide) and Dymelor (acetohexamide), which act to enhance the action or secretion of insulin; and the *biguanides*, including phenformin (DBI) which acts on the metabolic processes to decrease resistance to insulin action. These agents were used very widely in the 1960s, especially in older patients before it was generally appreciated that elevation of blood sugar appears to be an accompaniment of the ageing process and does not always need treatment. It was often found that these drugs were not useful for true insulin-dependent diabetics, but only for maturity-onset diabetics.

long-term effectiveness in question

In the 1960s, a large study of these drugs was undertaken to see if they were indeed more effective and safer than diet alone and insulin and diet. The results of the study have been the source of a great controversy in medicine since their publication. The study suggested that the drugs were no more, and possibly less, effective in preventing the long-term complications (stroke, heart attack, and arteriosclerosis) of diabetes than other traditional therapy. Many have criticized the design of the study and its findings are still argued, but it did cause many physicians to look critically at their prescription of these drugs and to generally limit use to a select group of persons who could not (or would not) control their diet and/or could not take or did not require insulin. The *biguanides* (phenformin) have been particularly criticized. Although effective in lowering blood sugar, they are also associated with producing a special complication called lactic acidosis, which requires more careful scrutiny by the physician. In general these drugs are used as therapy in addition to a well-regulated diet. In the absence of food, they can also cause a low blood sugar or hypoglycemia. Recently the government announced that it planned to ask for an orderly withdrawal of DBI from the market.

Listed below are some of the commonly prescribed drugs for diabetes. Those with an asterisk are individually described in Part III.

DBI*	NPH Insulin	Tolinase*
DBI-TD	Orinase*	
Diabinese*	regular insulin	

Oral contraceptives

how oral
contraceptives
work

Oral contraceptives have been taken by women in the United States since 1960. Although there are several types of contraceptive pill, the most common and most reliable is the type containing a combination of two synthetic female hormones, an *estrogen* and a *progestogen*. This combination-type pill, if taken regularly as directed, is almost 100% effective in preventing pregnancy.

The female menstrual cycle is regulated by several hormones and by interactions between these hormones. Among them are estrogen and progesterone (to which the synthetic progestogens are related) which are produced in the ovaries. The production of these hormones and of the ovum, or egg, released by an ovary each month, is stimulated by hormones from the pituitary gland, located at the base of the brain. Once the supply of ovarian hormones reaches a certain level, the supply of the pituitary hormones is depressed, working in a feedback system.

The minute amounts of additional estrogen supplied by oral contraceptives inhibit the production by the pituitary of the hormone that stimulates the growth, in the ovary, of the follicle containing the egg. The progestogen inhibits another pituitary hormone that triggers ovulation – the release of the egg. With no ovulation taking place, conception is impossible.

If by some remote chance an egg is produced, additional safeguards will stop a pregnancy. The progestogen contained in the pill has the effect of thickening the mucus in the cervical canal so that sperm cannot enter the uterus. Yet another function of the pill is to alter the lining of the uterus so that it would not be receptive to a fertilized egg in any case.

The estrogen-progestogen pill is taken for 21 days (sometimes a day more or less, according to the brand), starting on the fifth day of the menstrual cycle. (The first day of bleeding is counted as day 1). The pill is then stopped for a week. Within a few days of stopping the pill, menstruation begins. The amount of bleeding may be less than in a normal period, a fact which explains why women on the pill are less likely to suffer from iron deficiency than women who do not take the pill. Many women who have had irregular periods in the past may experience improvement in regularity, and some women with acne find that the condition improves after they begin taking the pill.

Women taking the combined estrogen-progestogen pill have reported a variety of side effects, including increased weight, depression, reduced sexual desire, cramps in the legs, and dryness in the vagina. If contact lenses are used, after use of the pill for several months the eyes can become dryer and more sensitive to the lenses. Each individual may react differently to different contraceptives. A woman's doctor may need to change the prescription once or twice to find one that minimizes the side effects. However, the body often needs a couple of months to adjust to this almost daily administration of extra hormones. Therefore, if side effects are not marked, it may be worthwhile to try a product for at least three cycles before changing to a different product.

There are many possible serious adverse effects of taking contraceptives. The most serious of these is the risk – a relatively low risk – of thrombosis. A thrombosis is the formation of a blood clot, usually in the deep veins of the leg or in the pelvis. If the clot moves to the lungs (where it is called a pulmonary embolism) it may cause death. In rare cases, another type of thrombosis may occur, in the blood vessels supplying the brain, to produce a stroke. In women over the age of 35, the risk of side effects is sufficiently large for many doctors to recommend alternate methods. These effects include gallbladder disease, and heart attacks (especially in heavy smokers).

Although the theory has not been conclusively proved, it is now believed that the estrogen in the pill may be the cause of this risk. Accordingly, doctors now tend to prescribe contraceptives containing the minimum effective dose of estrogen – 0.05 micrograms or less, although whether this does in fact decrease the risk is not yet clearly proven.

Some women, however, are at risk from taking any amount of additional estrogen. These include women who have had a thrombosis, those with some heart conditions, and those with past or present liver disease. For these women, another kind of contraceptive may be prescribed. One possible alternative is a pill containing only a progestogen. This pill is taken every day, instead of just for three weeks of the cycle, and it must be taken at the same time every day, whereas the estrogen-progestogen pill is effective even if 36 hours elapse between taking one pill and the next. The effectiveness of the progestogen pill depends mainly on its building up the sperm-deflecting mucus in the cervical canal; it apparently does not prevent ovulation. Even if the pill is taken every 24 hours, there is still a slightly greater risk of pregnancy than with a pill containing estrogen and a progestin. There are also some side effects, notably irregular and heavy periods.

A third type of contraceptive, the sequential type, is no longer prescribed in the United States. Each packet of sequential contraceptives contained some estrogen-only pills, to be taken on the first 15 days of the cycle, and some combined estrogen-progestogen pills to be taken on the following five to seven days.

precautions

All women should have a complete physical examination before starting the pill so that subsequent measurements, such as blood pressure, can be compared with the original ones. The leaflets provided with packets of pills explain the symptoms that you may observe while taking the pill and distinguish between those that are minor and those that should be reported to your doctor. For example, any increase in the frequency of headaches or pains in the legs or chest should be reported. The pill is stopped if your blood pressure rises, if vision becomes disturbed, or if migraine or jaundice develops. Although many women become pregnant soon after stopping the pill, a few have experienced difficulty. This difficulty is unrelated to the length of time the woman was taking the pill; it seems rather to be more common among women who started menstruating relatively late and had irregular periods. After a few months the reproductive organs and the pituitary gland will, in most cases, have adjusted to the loss of the extra hormones and will begin once more to function normally.

Listed below are some of the commonly prescribed oral contraceptives. Those with an asterisk are individually described in Part III.

Brevicon	Norinyl 1/50 21*	Ortho Novum
Demulen 21*	Norinyl 1/80 21	1/80 21*
Enovid	Norlestrin 21*	Ovral*
Loestrin	Nor. QD	Ovral 28*
Lo-Ovral*	Ortho-Novum*	Ovulen 21*
Micronor	Ortho-Novum	
Modicon	1/50 21*	

Estrogens and progestogens used in hormone therapy

menopause –
what is it and why
does it occur?

Although the oral contraceptives have enjoyed wide use for the last decade or so, female hormones also have been widely used in other circumstances, the most common being estrogen for treatment of postmenopausal symptoms. For example, Premarin, an estrogen preparation marketed almost exclusively for this purpose, is one of the most frequently prescribed drugs of any type. The wisdom of this widespread use is now being questioned, due to increased awareness of potential problems with long term use of the estrogens. Clearly-written brochures on the benefits and risks of such medication have been ordered by the government to be given with each prescription. This leaflet should be carefully read. If you have any further questions, discuss them fully with your doctor.

The female menopause is a period of time occurring between the mid-40s to early 50s when the ovaries begin to lose their ability to produce estrogens and progesterone. Thus ovulation and menstrual periods usually become irregular, less frequent, and finally cease. As the level of female hormones decreases, the feedback system through the brain and pituitary results in increased levels of the tropic hormones, FSH and LH. This process may occur over months to years. The same situation occurs, but more abruptly, when ovaries are removed surgically. The symptoms, which may or may not occur, are believed to be related to those changing levels of hormone in the blood.

The symptoms experienced in the menopause vary considerably in frequency, severity and duration. In addition to changes in menstrual periods, there are often symptoms of "hot flushes" or flushing, depression or irritability, and mood changes, especially in the early stages. As menopause progresses, there are reduced secretions in the vagina, which may produce irritation during intercourse and predispose to bladder irritation. Approximately 25% of women (usually white women) experience loss of bone (called osteoporosis) and may be more susceptible to fractures, especially of the spine.

wide use under
challenge

It has been common practice in the United States until very recently to give estrogen to almost all women with menopausal symptoms. This practice has recently been strongly challenged by the findings that use of the estrogens in this way increases the risk of cancer of the uterus, and a considerable controversy has arisen.

The arguments in favor of continued therapy contend that estrogens can markedly improve the quality of life of a women beset with hot flushes and mood changes, and most importantly, prevent spinal fractures, which may have crippling potential.

The arguments against have primarily cited the fairly well established increased risk of cancer of the uterus, and the potential for adverse cardiovascular effects such as thrombophlebitis and the risk of heart attack or stroke, which have been reported in older oral contraceptive users. It is also noted that the risk of osteoporosis is limited to only a certain proportion of women.

As yet, no simple answer has come out of this controversy, but it has served to stimulate more individualized therapy, which is desirable in any case. For example, many women, especially later in menopause, will have essentially no symptoms except dryness of the vagina. This is most easily relieved by local hormone therapy in an estrogen-containing vaginal cream. Although some estrogen may get into the body, the amounts are small, yet can entirely remove the symptoms.

It is generally felt that estrogen therapy in the menopause should be directed at relieving specific symptoms, such as hot flushes, or preventing specific problems such as osteoporosis. In young women with surgical removal of the ovaries, treatment is usually begun and continued to the usual time of menopause. The goal is to gradually decrease the dose and eventually discontinue the drug in both normal women and those who have had surgical menopause. An exception may be in those predisposed to osteoporosis, but this also remains controversial. It should be considerably clarified when better methods of measuring bone changes for early osteoporosis are found.

Estrogen therapy for postmenopausal symptoms is usually given in a cyclic fashion, that is, for three to four weeks, followed by a week off the drug, since this somewhat resembles a normal cyclic sequence and it may be less likely to predispose to uterine cancer if taken in this way. Common estrogen preparations used include Premarin, conjugated estrogens, and Estinyl. Some physicians will add a progesterone-like drug at the end of the cycle, to more closely resemble the normal cycle, but the real value of this remains unclear.

other uses of
estrogens

Estrogens are also used for other purposes. For example, they can be used to regulate irregular menstrual cycles, treat a disease called endometriosis and prevent pregnancy after rape (DES has been approved for this use). They are also used in two specific types of cancer therapy: cancer of the breast in certain postmenopausal women and cancer of the prostate in men.

Estrogens may have a variety of side effects and these are discussed in detail in the section on Oral Contraceptives. In general, they may cause weight gain, breast enlargement, some gastrointestinal distress, and on a longer term basis, they may predispose to gallbladder disease, blood clots in the legs and other circulatory problems. Because of the many effects, the pros and cons of estrogen therapy should always be discussed with the doctor and a regular exam, including breast check and Pap (Papanicolou) smear should be done every 6 to 12 months after stopping therapy.

progesterone,
the lesser-known
female hormone

Progesterone is the other major female hormone, but it has received much less publicity than the estrogen hormones. Progesterone and progesterone-like drugs, called progestogens, are similar in chemical structure to estrogens but they have somewhat different actions and are thought to have many fewer side effects than estrogens. This fact has stimulated some interest in the progestogen-only birth control pills (Miconor, Nor-Q.D. and Ovrette) but they are somewhat less effective in preventing pregnancy and have caused bleeding between cycles. Progesterone has also been incorporated into an intrauterine device (IUD), the Progestasert, but although it may be more effective than the IUD alone, the fact that it must be reinserted periodically has limited its use.

The other uses of progesterone are relatively specialized, primarily to treat abnormalities of the menstrual cycle, or cancer of the breast or uterus. Very rarely, progesterone is used to treat severe lung disease, as it does stimulate breathing. Preparations commonly used include progesterone, hydroxyprogesterone (Delalutin), medroxyprogesterone (Provera) and norethindrone (Norlutin).

Listed below are some of the commonly prescribed estrogens and progestogens used in hormone therapy. Those marked with an asterisk are individually described in Part III.

DES   Premarin*   Provera*
Estradiol

Steroids or cortisone-like drugs

Cortisone and related steroids resembling the hormones produced by the adrenal gland were introduced as "miracle" drugs for arthritis over 20 years ago. Subsequent experience reveals that the miracle had a very high price in the form of severe side effects. The cortisone-like drugs called corticosteroids, or simply steroids, have now gained wide use, but their proper role remains a subject of much controversy.

corticosteroid
hormones

The paired adrenal glands, located above each kidney, are stimulated by the hormone from the pituitary gland, ACTH, to secrete several steroid hormones: cortisone, hydrocortisone, and small amounts of male and female hormones, as well as other hormones. The corticosteroid hormones are classified in terms of two types of activity: glucocorticoid activity, or ability to affect sugar (glucose) metabolism; and mineralocorticoid activity, the ability to affect levels of the minerals sodium and potassium. Cortisone and hydrocortisone each exhibit some of both activities, which relate to their uses and side effects when used as medication. Many synthetic steroid hormones are produced that have similar activity to the natural hormones, cortisone and hydrocortisone, and, as in the case of prednisone, are more frequently used.

The corticosteroid hormones are used both as replacement therapy when the adrenal glands are not functioning (as in Addison's disease) and in higher doses for drug therapy in a variety of diseases. In replacement therapy, the naturally occurring hormones are most commonly used. In drug therapy, such synthetic corticosteroids as prednisone, methylprednisolone (Medrol) or triamcinolone (Kenalog) are used, partly because of their lower mineralocorticoid effect resulting in fewer problems of salt retention, edema and potassium loss.

broad spectrum
of activity

Corticosteroids have a broad spectrum of effects on the body, some of which can be very helpful in treating diseases, and some of which can cause equally severe unwanted side effects and reactions. The primary useful effects are associated with the glucocorticoid activity. They include suppression of inflammation (redness and swelling of an area), which is useful in such diverse diseases as poison ivy and poison oak, ulcerative disease of the colon (ulcerative colitis) and various types of acute arthritis.

Other effects include a decrease in scar formation, a decrease in immunity (which although hazardous, is also useful in such conditions as preventing kidney transplant rejection). In many cases, corticosteroids are used without a clear understanding of exactly how they work, although they are clearly known to be successful. These drugs have nevertheless been used in a very wide variety of acute and chronic disease. The list is long: rheumatoid arthritis; certain collagen diseases such as lupus erythematosus; certain types of chronic hepatitis; such serious widespread skin diseases as psoriasis; acute severe bronchial asthma; and blood diseases such as leukemias. In addition, they have been tried for treating shock and certain neurological diseases such as multiple sclerosis, where their effectiveness is argued.

many serious
side effects

The many significant adverse effects of these hormones used in high doses are clearly related to both the dose and duration of time given. Thus, a few days of even relatively high-dose therapy will infrequently cause problems. But beyond one to two weeks, problems invariably begin to appear. The glucocorticoids, in excess dose, usually cause a variety of metabolic changes. So, for example, the blood sugar often increases (which can bring out diabetes in those predisposed), and the body fat deposits become gradually redistributed (so the face often gets rounded, called a moon face, and fat is often deposited on the back of the neck, called a buffalo hump, and in the abdominal area). There is usually a weight gain, although this is partly due to the mineralocorticoid effects of salt and water retention. The decreased immunity, although useful in preventing rejection of kidney transplants, can also increase susceptibility to many types of infection, such as tuberculosis, or fungus infections. The suppression of scar formation, although useful in some settings, can also contribute to bruising easily, and to tissues that are thin and heal poorly. Corticosteroids make the protective mucous lining the stomach thinner and this is believed by many experts to predispose to peptic ulcers and bleeding. This is the reason antacids are frequently given along with steroid therapy. These hormones also affect calcium metabolism and over a long period of time weaken the bone structure and predispose to fractures, especially in the back or vertebral spine. There are also effects on the brain, so that persons receiving moderate doses (for example, 15 mg – 25 mg of prednisone per day) may feel in a better mood. Higher doses often produce mental symptoms such as hallucinations, but these are reversible by decreasing the dose.

Those corticosteroids with mineralocorticoid effect – hydrocortisone and prednisone for example – can also cause salt and water retention (and thus swelling of the hands and feet) and loss of the mineral potassium, which can cause weakness. The frequent practice of treating this edema with diuretics (see Diuretics) may compound the problem as they cause potassium loss.

It is apparent that because of these adverse effects, corticosteroids used other than locally or for short periods (less than 7–10 days) are ideally used only when less toxic drugs are ineffective and/or therapy is life-saving. A final condition further emphasizes this need for caution.

an additional problem – and a way out

As in the case for other hormones, a high level of adrenocorticosteroid hormone signals to the master gland, the pituitary, to decrease release of ACTH, the tropic hormone that stimulates the adrenal gland to produce the steroid hormone (see Hormonal Drugs). If a steroid is given at high levels for a long time, the adrenal gland gradually shrinks due to a lack of stimulation, and after a time stops working. Therefore, once corticosteroids have been taken for longer periods (greater than two to three weeks) they must be gradually withdrawn to allow the adrenal gland to recover. This withdrawal can be done in a variety of ways. If steroids, such as prednisone, have been taken for months or years, it may take several months to completely discontinue the drug safely. A person on corticosteroids for long periods should wear appropriate identification since in time of stress (an auto accident or surgery), they may need extra steroids to prevent serious complications.

Fortunately, it was discovered several years ago that in many cases it is possible to give certain corticosteroids every other day and get almost the same beneficial effects but avoid most of the side effects noted above plus the shrinkage and loss of function of the person's adrenal glands. This method has obviously offered advantages and has been very useful in certain diseases, especially in children. In other types of diseases, such as some cases of severe rheumatoid arthritis, this method has not been successful.

Corticosteroids are given by mouth, by injection, as enemas (for ulcerative colitis), in the eyes for inflammation, and are applied to the skin (steroid creams and ointments are one of the most frequently used dermatological drugs). Recently, they have been used as aerosols (Vanceril, or beclomethasone) in treatment of chronic asthma. They are used locally by injection into joints, or into other inflamed areas such as large acne lesions. The overall principle has been to use corticosteroids locally when possible, and in high doses for short periods. The pituitary gland hormone, ACTH or adrenocorticotropic hormone, which stimulates the adrenal gland to produce steroids, is sometimes administered by injection in place of the corticosteroid hormones. It also is used to test the adrenal gland for its level of functioning. Except when used as a test, it is usually less preferable than the actual hormone. In summary, corticosteroid hormones have occasional use as replacement therapy but extremely wide use as drug therapy for many ailments of many organs. The problems with the drug emphasize the critical need for careful cost benefit analysis whenever their long-term use is considered.

Listed below are some of the commonly prescribed steroids or cortisone-like drugs. Those marked with an asterisk are individually described in Part III.

Decadron   Medrol*   prednisone*

Stimulants and drugs for weight loss

Excess body fat, or obesity, is a common problem in our overfed Western society. Most of us eat more and exercise less than we should, and the result is often excess pounds. Severe obesity, besides being unattractive, may be dangerous. Many doctors now believe that the obese person has a decreased life expectancy and a greater than average chance of contracting diabetes, gallstones, cardiovascular disorders and orthopedic problems – although the extent to which obesity helps to cause these disorders is debated.

The possible health hazards of obesity and the desire to be more attractive induce millions of overweight people to try reducing techniques of various kinds. A seemingly endless number of treatments for obesity have been announced in the popular press, each heralded as the ideal method. These include radical diets consisting of only a few specific foods or liquids; various kinds of psychotherapy, including aversion therapy and hypnosis; medical treatments using hormones and other drugs) and even surgical procedures such as wiring the jaw shut, removing part of the intestine, or removing the fat itself in certain areas.

Some overweight people believe that their problem has a glandular cause. Actually, glandular disorders account for only a small fraction of all cases of obesity. A sudden increase in appetite or weight is sometimes associated with decreased thyroid function or adrenal gland disorder, or some other endocrine disturbance. But the great majority of overweight people acquire their excess pounds gradually through habits of overeating that often begin in childhood. The overeating may have a psychological cause, and in such cases some form of psychotherapy may help the person to get at the root of his problem.

The only method of losing weight safely and maintaining the reduced weight is to reduce one's intake of calories by eating less and adhering to a balanced diet low in starches, sweets, and fats. "Crash" diets or radical diets may achieve a sudden weight loss, but they fail to establish a healthy pattern of food intake needed for maintaining the reduced weight. This kind of diet is almost invariably followed by an overeating spree and, consequently, a weight increase.

Many drugs have been used in the treatment of obesity. None have been shown to be consistently effective in producing long-lasting weight loss. Some are very hazardous.

Among the most widely-promoted weight-loss products are the bulk fillers and expanders. These are available over the counter, usually in the form of cookies or candies. They generally contain methyl-cellulose, a compound which expands in the stomach to give a sensation of fullness. These drugs are safe and do help to prevent constipation. They also help to curb appetite by creating a full-stomach feeling. They are customarily taken before meals with water. Whether their effect is due to curbing the appetite, or due to the psychological effect of just doing "something" is not clear – possibly it's a combination of both.

A group of drugs frequently prescribed in reducing programs are the anorexiants. They include the amphetamines and other drugs which resemble amphetamines. Their name, anorexiants, is derived from the medical term anorexia, which means loss of appetite; and they can cause a loss of appetite for a period of a few days to several weeks. It is important to realize that the drug itself has no direct effect on body weight; what it does is to stimulate the central nervous system in such a way as to make you want less food. Soon, however, the body will develop a tolerance for the drug, and as the appetite-suppressant effect wears off, the person taking the drug will resume his or her former eating habits – unless he or she has, in the meantime, resolutely established a restricted diet. In other words, an anorexiant might help to *launch* a diet, but it will not do the *work* of dieting for the person hoping to lose weight.

The use of these drugs has more serious drawbacks. Because they tend to make the user feel alert and full of energy (although they make some people nervous and jittery), he or she may be tempted to increase the dose as time goes on, in order to regain the original euphoric effect – which the original dose no longer provides. A habit of dependence is quickly established. Side effects of the anorexiants include rapid heartbeat and increased blood pressure. These characteristics make them hazardous for people suffering from heart ailments or hypertension.

The amphetamines are particularly dangerous in terms of their addictive potential. Widespread abuse of these drugs in recent years has led to their being classified by Federal law as restricted drugs. The number of amphetamines prescribed by doctors and the number kept in stock by pharmacists must be reported and must not exceed certain limits. By law, package inserts on amphetamines must bear the following warning:

Amphetamines have a high potential for abuse. They should thus be tried only in weight reduction programs for patients in whom alternative therapy has been ineffective. Administration of amphetamines for prolonged periods of time in obesity may lead to drug dependence and must be avoided.

Diuretics are drugs that rid the body of excess water, and in the process cause it to lose some weight. Women who have been prescribed a diuretic to relieve premenstrual swelling and discomfort sometimes use the drug to help them reduce, and some doctors prescribe a diuretic in the first few weeks of a weight-reducing program. However, the long-term use of a diuretic has no effect on fat. The use of diuretics in reducing programs can be hazardous, because they deprive the body of necessary minerals, such as potassium. They have no place in legitimate weight reducing programs.

Preparations containing the thyroid hormone are often used inappropriately by weight control clinics because they speed up the metabolism of the cells and so cause the body to burn up more calories. This is because when the thyroid gland is overactive and produces excess hormone a weight loss will occur, despite an increase in appetite. Other effects of this condition, called hyperthyroidism, are nervousness, irritability, diarrhea, and increased heart rate. The same symptoms may be produced by a large dose of the hormone. If a person has been taking a thyroid preparation and suddenly stops taking it, he or she may experience a temporary state of hypothyroidism, or abnormally low thyroid activity, with its accompanying symptoms of fatigue, sleepiness, and sluggishness. Thus, weight reduction with thyroid preparations can be hazardous. These drugs should be used only when the person is suffering from hypothyroidism and not for simple weight control. (See Drugs for Thyroid Disorders.)

Another hormone often used in reducing clinics in the U.S. is human chorionic gonadotropin (HCG) a product of the placenta similar to a pituitary hormone. Its weight-reducing properties – if any – have not been clearly established. Most clinics giving HCG injections also put their patients on a very low calorie diet, which will in itself cause a weight loss. When the treatment is stopped the patient often quickly regains the lost weight.

To sum up, drugs have very limited usefulness in weight reduction programs. A balanced, low-calorie diet is the only sure, safe way to lose weight.

Listed below are some of the commonly prescribed drugs for weight loss. Those with an asterisk are individually described in Part III.

amphetamines	Dexamyl	Ritalin*
Dexedrine	Ionamin*	Tenuate*

Drugs for asthma and lung disease

how the lungs work

To understand how drugs for lung disease work, we must first look at the way the lungs themselves work. Each lung contains a system of tubes called bronchi and smaller tubes called bronchioles that branch out from the trachea, or windpipe. The bronchioles end in clusters of tiny sacs called alveoli. The thin walls of the alveoli contain minute blood vessels which absorb the oxygen we breathe in. Red blood cells carry the oxygen to other parts of the body, and they also bring back to the lungs the waste product carbon dioxide, which is released when we exhale. Since this oxygen-carbon dioxide exchange is essential for life, it is vital that the airways of the lungs be kept open.

constriction of the airways

In some respiratory diseases – notably asthma, but also in some cases of "reactive" bronchitis and emphysema – there is constriction of muscles around the bronchioles, causing them to contract and so restrict the exchange of air. The cause of this constriction varies from one person to another. It may be a substance to which the person is allergic, such as pollen or cat fur; it may be inhalation of cold air or of an irritant such as cigarette smoke; or it may be emotional stress. The resulting bronchoconstriction is indicated by the symptom of wheezing – a high-pitched whistling sound caused by the air trying to get through partially constricted airways.

Narrowing of the airways also occurs in bronchitis, a disease in which repeated infection of the bronchial tubes causes scarring and narrowing of the tubes. In emphysema the lung tissues lose their elastic quality, so that when the person breathes out, some bronchioles may close and air may be trapped in the lungs. Unfortunately, because both emphysema and chronic bronchitis bring about a permanent change in the small bronchial tubes, neither condition responds as effectively to drug therapy as does asthma, in which the constriction of the bronchial tubes is due to temporary spasm.

how bronchodilators work

Most drugs used to open the airways of the lungs act on the muscles in the bronchial tubes and are called bronchodilators. These bronchodilators include epinephrine, theophylline, Tedral, Marax, and Isuprel. It is now believed that most of these drugs achieve their results by regulating the amount of a hormone-like substance called cyclic AMP in the bronchial muscles.

An increase of cyclic AMP in these muscles causes them to relax. When the substance is used up, the muscle tends to constrict again. One group of bronchodilators acts to increase the production of cyclic AMP and so relax the muscles. These are drugs related to adrenaline (epinephrine), such as ephedrine, Brethine, and Alupent. If these drugs are used continually, the body may develop resistance, or tolerance to their effects, and they will become less useful. They can also have adverse effects including an increased heart rate, palpitations, high blood pressure, trembling, and dizziness.

Another group of bronchodilator drugs act in a preventive way by inhibiting the breakdown of cyclic AMP in the bronchial muscles. This preventive action has the same result as the increased production of cyclic AMP caused by the first group of drugs; it raises the level of cyclic AMP and so helps the muscles to relax. This second group of drugs includes theophylline and others resembling it. Adverse effects of these drugs include rapid heart rate, loss of appetite, nausea, and vomiting.

Bronchodilators can be taken in a number of ways. Most of them are available in inhalers, which permit small droplets of the drug to be inhaled through the mouth into the bronchial tubes. This is probably the quickest, but not necessarily the most efficient way to get the drug where it is needed. Bronchodilators are also given orally, by injection, and even as rectal suppositories, in the case of theophylline.

Another group of drugs acts by preventing bronchoconstriction from occurring in the first place. For example, in the case of allergic asthma – asthma caused by an allergic reaction – some antihistamines and other drugs such as Intal will block the constrictive action of histamine on the muscles and reduce the severity of an attack. However, they are not effective against all substances causing an allergic reaction.

In cases of severe asthma one of the cortisone-like drugs such as prednisone may be prescribed. These drugs are thought to act partly to increase the effect of the bronchodilator drugs and also possibly to prevent recurrent attacks of the disease. They belong to a group of drugs called steroids. Prednisone is usually taken orally, either for a short period with a dose tapering off gradually or on a long term basis in a low dosage. Another type of steroid recently put on the market is administered by inhaler and is called Vanceril.

It is important to remember that the immediate causes of bronchoconstriction can vary considerably. A person can be breathing completely normally, and then come in contact with something that causes his bronchial airways to close suddenly. Naturally, the wheezing and difficult breathing which result can be alarming, and it is important that he be prepared for it – by learning from his doctor how to use the drugs that have been prescribed for him, how long they take to act, and exactly how much and how often they should by used (excessive use of either inhalors or oral drugs may cause more harm than good and make subsequent therapy more difficult).

Listed below are some of the commonly prescribed drugs for asthma and lung disease. Those with an asterisk are individually described in Part III.

Aarane	Elixophyllin*	Tedral*
Alupent	Intal	theophylline
Bricanyl	Marax*	Vanceril
Bronkosol	Quibron*	

Drugs to treat infections

what is an infection?

Simply stated, an infection is the invasion of the body by parasites, including bacteria, viruses, protozoa, or fungus. These organisms cause infections that can be local, such as a boil on the skin or pneumonia in the lungs, or general, as is common with typhoid, mumps or malaria, where many parts of the body are affected. The symptoms and damage resulting from an infection are caused both by the organism's invasion of tissue, and the response of the body's defense system. The most common signs of infection are inflammation (pain, heat, redness, swelling and pus production), and often fever.

Not all microorganisms produce infections, and even those that can, called pathogenic organisms, do not do so all the time. Those bacteria better at breaching the body's defense mechanisms are more likely to cause disease and are described as virulent. At this end of the spectrum are the bacteria that cause cholera and typhoid fever; they almost always cause a severe infection if they enter an unimmunized person. At the other end of the scale are bacteria such as those found in yoghurt (*Lactobacillus bulgaricus*) which rarely cause infection. It is also true that the fewer bacteria present, the lower the likelihood of infection. This is why it is advisable to cleanse and cover open wounds or cuts. Location of the bacteria also affects their ability to cause infection. Under normal circumstances, with good standards of hygiene, the bacteria in the air, on the skin and in the mouth and intestine, are harmless. Individual response to potential invaders differs according to the state of the body's defense mechanisms, including natural antibodies and those that result from vaccination, plus white blood cells called phagocytes, which "eat" foreign organisms. When infection does occur, more phagocytes are produced and travel through the bloodstream to the site.

when do we get infections?

Some individuals have a decreased resistance to infection because of frequent bouts with diseases or due to certain drugs that reduce the effectiveness of the body's defense system. Included in this group are persons with kidney or other organ transplants, and those receiving anticancer or cortisone-like drugs. Exposure of such individuals even to small number of pathogenic organisms may cause infection.

methods of prevention

In summary, whether infection occurs depends on the balance between these factors: the virulence, numbers and location of the organism; and, most importantly, the resistance of the individual. These factors provide a strong basis for the principles of prevention and treatment.

Prevention of infection may involve a variety of measures:

– Lowering the number of microorganisms by keeping the skin clean, using antiseptics (agents to prevent the growth of microorganisms), and by prophylactic use of antibiotics before surgery.

– Decreasing exposure to pathogenic organisms through quarantine, isolation, or simply avoiding infected persons.

– Increasing the individual immunity by vaccination.

...and treatment

Treatment of infection through medication aims to decrease the number of microorganisms or eliminate them without significantly harming the host, that is the infected person. By this means, the host can recover or continue to fight the few remaining organisms. Treating infections in people with very low resistance is much more difficult, and direct aids to the body's defenses, such as extra white blood cells, may be necessary.

Some infections are easier to treat than others. Those caused by bacteria, such as strep throat (a streptococcal infection), bladder infection, and bacterial pneumonia, are often readily treated with antimicrobial drugs. In contrast, most viral infections such as measles, mumps, herpes simplex (cold sores), encephalitis, and the common cold, are either difficult or impossible to treat, although some symptoms, for example fever, can be treated. Between these extremes are infections caused by fungi and parasites, which are sometimes easily treated and sometimes not – these are discussed later.

Antibiotics: their sources and functions

Medication used to treat infections caused by microorganisms (microbes) are called antimicrobial drugs, among which are antibiotics and sulfa drugs (discussed later). Antibiotics are themselves produced by microorganisms; they can be obtained from molds or other microorganisms and are then purified or modified for therapeutic use. For centuries, certain moldy materials were known to be useful in treating local infections such as boils. But not until 1928 did Alexander Fleming discover that the mold *Penicillium notatum*, growing accidently in a bacterial culture, could kill bacteria. Following this chance observation, the active substance was identified and called penicillin. But not until 1941 was penicillin tested in humans – this date marks the beginning of the present antibiotic era of drug treatment.

Antibiotics are among the most frequently prescribed drugs today after sedatives and tranquilizers; they account for up to one-third of some hospital pharmacy budgets. They can be used both to treat, and prevent, bacterial infection but they are essentially ineffective against viruses and only effective against some parasites and fungi. Antibiotics may be bactericidal (killing the bacteria) or bacteristatic (stopping bacterial multiplication). They act in conjunction with the body's defenses to overcome infection, but in serious infections, their timely help is essential to redress the balance in favor of the host and provide a chance to recover.

Some antibiotics are very specific; they kill some kinds of organisms, but not others. These are classified by the type of bacteria they affect; in turn, bacteria are classed by whether they can be dyed with a particular microscopic stain, Gram stain. Those that take up the blue dye are called Gram positive (such as Streptococcus, which causes strep throat); those that do not are called Gram negative (Salmonella, which causes food poisoning) and appear red under the microscope. Bacteria are also divided by shape into cocci (round) and bacilli (rod-like). An antibiotic that is effective against more than one such category, for instance Gram positive and Gram negative bacilli, is described as a broad spectrum antibiotic.

to test or not to test?

Infections that occur commonly, such as strep throat, local infections of the hands and feet, or gonorrhea, are known to be sensitive to particular antibiotics. For example, strep throat is almost always treated with penicillin, except in persons who are sensitive to penicillin, when erythromycin is usually used. But in many infections, bacteria are collected from an infected source, such as the throat or urine, cultured, and tested for their sensitivity to a range of antibiotics (a procedure often abbreviated to C and S). In this way, the antibiotics most likely to be effective can be identified. In chronic infections, as in the bladder, sensitivity testing is also very helpful because the bacteria may become resistant to the antibiotic normally used.

administration

Antibiotics are given systemically by injection and orally, as well as locally on the skin, in the eye and other places. Many common antibiotics, such as tetracycline, are not well absorbed into the blood stream if taken with food, so most oral antibiotics should be taken on an empty stomach. When taken orally, many of these drugs may cause diarrhea, because the antibiotic affects some of the bacteria in the gut. This effect is not usually a major problem, but in certain cases, for instance with clindamycin (Cleocin), diarrhea can be a serious problem and any occurence should be discussed with a doctor.

seeing the treatment through

Antibiotics for treating infections are usually taken for at least five days, and more often for eight to ten days. Completion of the course of treatment is most important, even though one often feels better, with a normal temperature, after two or three days. If the medication is not all taken, any surviving, temporarily subdued bacteria may later cause a relapse. Worse, the bacteria may develop a partial immunity to that particular antibiotic making future treatment more difficult.

antibiotic groups

Specific antibiotics and their characteristics are discussed under their individual names in Part III, but the common antibiotics can usefully be considered in groups, for several reasons:

– Antibiotics in the same group often act in a similar way.

– If an allergy or immunity exists to one antibiotic in a group, it will likely transfer to other antibiotics in the same group.

– In some cases, the major difference within a group

91

may be cost: if this consideration arises, checking with your physician may be worthwhile.

The major, most commonly prescribed antibiotics are described in this book, though in some cases only the generic forms have been fully dealt with since the brand names are identical.

Antimicrobial drugs other than antibiotics

sulfonamides
(sulfa drugs)

Certain antimicrobial drugs cannot be obtained from molds or other organisms. Apart from the means of production, the reasons for using these drugs, their mode of action, and the duration of therapy are the same as for antibiotics. Sulfa drugs (properly called sulfonamides), first used clinically in 1935, were derived from dyes produced in Germany in the early 1900s.

Sulfa drugs enjoyed wide use against bacterial infections and provided the first effective method of treating certain diseases, such as gonorrhea and bacterial meningitis. But for a variety of reasons, their use declined with the advent of penicillin and the subsequent development of other antibiotics, such as chloramphenicol (Chloromycetin) and chlortetracycline (Aureomycin). Nevertheless, many sulfa drugs (notably Gantrisin), are still widely used in the effective treatment of bladder and urinary tract infections.

Sulfa drugs, including co-trimoxazole, are usually taken in the form of rather large pills washed down with lots of water, since the drug has a slight tendency to recrystallize, which could cause damage in the kidney. This precautionary measure is always important, although the problem is less common with some newer sulfonamides.

other chemicals
with
antibacterial
action

In the late 1960s, an unrelated antimicrobial agent (trimethoprim) was found to increase the effectiveness of sulfonamides. Accordingly, trimethoprim plus a sulfonamide in a combination called co-trimoxazole (Bactrim, Septra) has recently been introduced. This combination drug reduces the chance that bacteria will become resistant to the antimicrobial action, a problem that has been quite common with sulfa drugs. Overcoming this resistance makes co-trimethoprim especially useful in treating chronic bladder infections, but the product seems to have a broad range of effective uses. Another frequently prescribed major antibacterial drug is the antiseptic nitrofurantoin, or Macrodantin. It is used to treat protracted urinary diseases that do not respond to other medication.

Antiviral drugs

Very few drugs are effective in treating viral infections.

The only preparation with any wide use in idoxuridine (Stoxil), and that only for a particular type of eye infection. Considerable research is being carried out to find clinically useful antiviral agents, and hundreds of chemicals, both naturally produced and synthetic, are being tested. Unfortunately, many doctors are under pressure to "prescribe something" when patients come in with valid complaints, such as chest colds. Antibiotics are usually prescribed, although they have absolutely no effect on the virus.

Antifungal drugs

Fungal infections within the body are fortunately uncommon and are extremely difficult to treat, but those on the skin or nails, or in the vaginal region are susceptible to direct treatment. Such local fungal infections tend to persist or recur, and in many cases treatment must continue for lengthy periods. For example, griseofulvin, the oral antibiotic used to treat fungal nail infections, often needs to be taken for six months to a year. Tolnaftate (Tinactin), one of several antifungal drugs applied locally to treat common fungal infections of the skin, (athlete's foot), commonly needs to be used regularly for 10 to 14 days to assure success. Other antifungal drugs, including the antibiotic nystatin (Mycostatin), are discussed further in the chapter on Drugs for Skin and Local Disorders.

antitrichomonal drugs

One other often-prescribed antimicrobial drug deserves mention. Since its usefulness was discovered in 1960, metronidazole (Flagyl) has found an established place in the treatment of vaginal infections caused by the common protozoan Trichomonas. This is discussed further in the chapter on Drugs for Skin and Local Disorders. More recently, metronidazole has been found effective in other parasitic and bacterial infections.

Listed below are some of the commonly prescribed drugs to treat infections. Those with an asterisk are individually described in Part III.

Achromycin/V*	E.E.S.*	Keflin
Amcill*	E-Mycin*	Laratid*
Ampicillin*	Erythrocin*	Macrodantin*
Amoxil*	erythromycin*	Minocin*
Ancef	Gantanol*	Mycolog*
Azo Gantrisin*	Gantrisin*	Mycostatin
Bactrim	Garamycin*	Mysteclin-F*
Cefadyl	Ilosone*	Omnipen
Chloromycetin	Keflex *	Pediamycin*

penicillin G*	Principen	tetracycline*
penicillin VK*	Robitet*	V-Cillin-K*
Pentids*	Septra*	Vibramycin*
Pen-Vee-K*	sulfasoxisole	
Polycillin	Sumycin	

Drugs for coughs and colds

There are literally hundreds of drugs available by prescription or over-the-counter for treatment of the symptoms of colds and related problems such as hay fever and sinusitis. None of the drugs cures colds, or shortens their duration, but some can relieve the symptoms. Many of the drugs, especially combination products, are directed to some or all of the symptoms. Therefore, it is useful to define the symptoms and see how they can be relieved by the multitude of remedies.

what is a cold?

The common cold is undoubtedly man's most widespread affliction, a source of general inconvenience and loss of work. Unfortunately, partly due to the fact that colds are caused by viruses (and no drugs are known to cure most viral illnesses), the successful prevention, cure, or even shortening of colds, is somewhere in the future. The much publicized role of vitamin C in preventing or curing colds is still argued, but there is no need to discuss it further here. Likewise, the role of antibiotics such as penicillin, which have no effect on the true common cold due to a virus. For the present, therapy is aimed at relieving the very typical symptoms, which may vary in severity from person to person or from one episode to another.

Characteristically, the symptoms of a cold start with either the fairly sudden onset of sneezing and runny nose, or a tickling sensation or sore sensation at the back of the throat. This is sometimes followed by fever, headache, general aching, a husky voice or laryngitis, sore throat and often a few days later, a cough. The symptoms may continue for as long as 7 to 14 days. A closer look at the types of symptoms will clarify why certain drugs are included in the medications commonly used. It is important to note that certain other disorders, especially hay fever, vascular rhinitis or allergic sinusitis, have many similar symptoms and often are treated with the same drugs.

Sneezing and a runny nose, which is also stuffy, are

sneezing, runny
and stuffy nose
and sinus
congestion

usual symptoms of a cold, but also of hay fever or allergic rhinitis (affecting the nose) or sinusitis. These symptoms are due to the increased fluid and mucus production and swelling of the lining of the nose, and the sinuses – hollow cavities which branch out from inside the nose above and below the eyes. There are actually three kinds of drugs which are used to relieve these symptoms: (1) decongestants, (2) anticholinergic drugs, and (3) antihistamine drugs.

The sensations of a stuffy nose, blocked ears (due to swelling of the eustachian tubes extending from the back of the throat to the ears) and congested sinuses are due to swelling of mucous membranes in this area. The swelling in turn is due to dilation of blood vessels caused by either the cold or allergic reaction. Sometimes blood vessels will dilate from other causes, but that produces the same symptoms. Decongestants act to constrict the blood vessels, which decreases the swelling. These blood – vessel-constricting drugs, or vasoconstrictors, are found in the nasal sprays such as Afrin or Neo-Synephrine and are also found in many of the cough/cold medicines such as Actifed, Sudafed, Allerest, Dimetapp or Ornade. The common decongestant component of these mixtures includes such drugs as ephedrine, pseudoephedrine, phenylephrine, phenylpropanolamine, napthazoline, and oxymetazoline, to name a few. Most of these decongestants are effective, but they have some drawbacks. If they are used repeatedly, they begin to lose their effectiveness and greater amounts may be needed. Also, since they do cause constriction of all blood vessels in the body, they often raise the blood pressure and increase the heart rate somewhat. This is not usually a serious problem unless the person has high blood pressure or is taking drugs for high blood pressure, in which case it is worthwhile consulting a physician.

drugs for runny
nose and mucus
congestion

When the nose and sinuses are affected in a cold or allergy they respond by producing more fluid and mucus. If this is due to an allergy, it may involve the release of histamine. For this reason, antihistamine drugs such as methapyrilene, doxylamine, pyrilamine, brompheniramine, chlorpheniramine, and diphenhydramine are found in a variety of cough/cold medications and may be helpful in drying the secretions. However they also reduce natural bacteria barriers and cause drowsiness. In the absence of allergy, as in the common cold, secretions can be decreased if an anticholinergic drug, such as atropine or belladonna alkaloid is used. Since most antihistamine drugs also have anticholinergic effects, which enable them to work on the common cold, they are the drugs usually preferred. The majority of cough/cold preparations do have either antihistamines or anticholinergic drugs in them.

cough-suppressants versus expectorants

Most persons with a cold develop a cough, often several days later. A cough is essentially the rapid elimination of air from the lungs which produces a noise. This symptom is a protective reflex which occurs in all persons to clear the bronchial tube of any foreign material, including mucus. In some cases, the airways are simply irritated and the cough is a reflex response. Drugs for coughs may act in two separate and sometimes opposite ways: (1) to simply suppress coughing, or (2) to loosen or help liquify the mucus in the lungs, called an expectorant effect. The expectorant may both decrease or increase coughing! By increasing the amount of mucus it actually stimulates coughing, while, on the other hand, it can reduce coughing by decreasing irritation from drying mucus. Cough suppressants, for their part, can act either locally in the bronchial tubes to prevent irritation, or in the brain to prevent the cough reflex. Codeine is one of the most effective cough suppressants known, but other cough suppressants also include the non-narcotic drugs dextromethorphan (Romilar), and diphenhydramine, which is the antihistamine Benadryl. Although these medications are effective, the suppression of a protective cough which helps get rid of mucus and prevents obstruction is only indicated when coughing becomes repetitive and very bothersome. Coughs should only be suppressed for short periods.

The majority of cough medicines contain one or more drugs which are included for their expectorant effect – ability to liquify thick mucus or phlegm to help with its elimination. Drugs which are used for this effect include terpin hydrate, glyceryl guaiacolate, benzoin, camphor, menthol and iodides. Unfortunately, although the theory of expectorant action is good, it has been difficult to determine whether any of these drugs really functions in quite this way. Since the problem has been recently emphasized, prompting an FDA review of cough and cold medicines, it may be that this issue will be clarified in the near future. In the meantime, it is likely that most cough syrups with expectorants will continue to be used with the hope that they relieve some symptoms – although simply drinking adequate fluids may be sufficient to give the same expectorant effect. Whether the extra drug is worth the expense remains to be seen.

other cold symptoms: pain, fever

Not uncommonly, a patient afflicted with a cold will experience one to two days of feeling tired, and may have headache, muscle aches or back pains, which are fairly typical of most other infectious illnesses. The major useful additional drug for the cold sufferer is one which reduces the pains and fevers, if any. The most commonly used drugs, which in fact do both, are aspirin and acetaminophen (Tylenol). One or the other of these may also be included in some cough/cold medications such as Phenaphen with codeine. Frequently, these drugs (aspirin or acetaminophen) are the only ones really needed for treating most colds, taken with lots of fluids and adequate rest.

Listed below are some of the commonly prescribed drugs for coughs, colds and sinus allergies. Those with an asterisk are individually described in Part III.

Actifed*	Neosynephrine	Phenergan VC Ex.*
Actifed-C Ex.*	nasal spray	Phenergan VC Ex/
Afrin*	Novahistine-DH*	Codeine*
Ambenyl Ex.*	Novahistine Ex.*	Singlet*
Benylin Cough	Ornade*	Sudafed*
Syrup*	Phenergan Ex.*	Tuss-Ornade*
Drixoral*	Phenergan Ex/	
Naldecon*	Codeine*	

Antihistamines

a versatile drug

The term antihistamine refers to a class of drugs available over the counter or by prescription, which have a variety of uses. First, they are used to counteract some symptoms of allergic reactions such as stuffy nose or congested sinuses due to allergy or hay fever; they are often not very effective in allergic asthma. Antihistamines are also used to help relieve itching in skin eruptions, especially those due to allergy such as hives. Since they cause drowsiness, these preparations are also often used to treat anxiety, or as mild sleeping pills. Finally, they can act to decrease nausea and vertigo due to motion sickness, so some

97

antihistamines (such as Dramamine) are used for motion sickness.

three types of action

The numerous uses stem from the variety of pharmocologic effects that these drugs share. The most important is their ability to block the effects of histamine, a substance released by the body in allergic-type reactions. Histamine can cause nasal stuffiness, itching and redness of the skin, and local swelling. Antihistamines are more effective when used prior to, or in anticipation of, an allergic reaction, or when used in a continuing allergic reaction, as in hay fever or allergic sinusitis.

Antihistamines also cause varying degrees of drowsiness. The effect is sufficiently common so that certain antihistamines such as Atorax or Vistoril and Benadryl are used as anti-anxiety or sleeping medication. However in other situations, drowsiness comprises a major bothersome side effect, which can interfere with concentration, driving and operating machinery. Another unwanted effect of over-the-counter cough and cold remedies containing antihistamines which reduce nasal secretions is that they may do harm by drying the lining of the nose respiratory tract. Not only can this lower the body's defences against infection, but an actual increase of congestion can result.

Finally, antihistamines, especially Dramamine and Antivert, act on the brain to decrease nausea and vertigo associated with motion sickness and certain disorders of the inner ear, such as Meniere's syndrome.

Despite this wide assortment of effects, antihistamines are relatively safe drugs, bearing in mind that they can cause allergic reactions, that the drowsiness may be bothersome, and that the sedation is additive to other sedatives, tranquilizers and alcohol. Antihistamines are generally inexpensive, especially in single generic ingredient forms, but are somewhat more expensive in combinations such as Orinade or Dimetapp.

Listed below are some of the commonly prescribed antihistamines or antihistamine-containing drugs. Those with an asterisk are individually described in Part III.

Actifed*	Benadryl Cap./	chlorpheniramine
Actifed-C Ex.*	Tabs.*	Chlor-Trimeton
Ambenyl Ex.*	Benadryl Elixir*	Tabs.*
Antivert*	Benylin Cough	Dimetane Ex.*
Atarax*	Syrup*	Dimetane Ex.DC*

Dimetane Tabs.* Periactin* Polaramine Tabs.*
Dimetapp* Phenergan Ex.* Singlet*
Dramamine Phenergan Ex. Teldrin*
Drixoral* Codeine* Tuss Ornade*
Naldecon* Phenergan Vistaril*
Novahistine-DH* VC Ex.*
Novahistine Ex.* Phenergan
Ornade* VC Ex./Codeine

Vaccines

Vaccines are not medicines, but a discussion of vaccines has been included in this book since they are given to almost every individual in the United States at one time or another and are a vital part of maintaining good health.

Vaccines and antiserums are used to build immunity against infectious diseases caused by bacteria or viruses.

active and
passive
immunity

Two kinds of immunity can be produced. In active immunity, the vaccine stimulates the body to make antibodies against the bacteria, the toxins produced by bacteria, or the virus. If a person is then exposed to the infection, a protective mechanism already exists in the body to fight the disease. This immunity can last many years (as the 7 – 10 years with tetanus toxoid) or a very short time, as with influenza vaccines.

Passive immunity is obtained when the serum containing antibodies from another person or animal (called antiserum) is given after exposure to the infectious disease to prevent severe effects of the disease (as in rabies) or to counteract the toxin (as in botulism or tetanus). This type of immunity is very short in duration and is only given after the person has been exposed to the disease or toxin.

There are several types of vaccines. Some bacterial vaccines are made from small amounts of killed whole bacteria or from the toxins produced by bacteria (in which case the vaccine is called a toxoid). Vaccines for viral infections are commonly made from live viruses, which have been greatly modified in a laboratory so that they do not produce disease but do signal the body to produce antibodies to fight the harmful virus. This is why, in certain cases, mild symptoms are experienced, as when measles or mumps vaccine is given. In other cases, killed viruses are used.

There are some very general facts about vaccines or antiserums that are important to understand fully. In recent years, it has been found that some persons have failed to receive certain vaccines, such as measles, or polio, and this has resulted in some outbreaks of these diseases which might have been prevented. For this reason, it is very important for everyone to have a record of their immunizations.

The majority of virus vaccines are made from modified viruses which cause no disease. These include measles, mumps, rubella, polio and smallpox. However, persons who have low immunity, such as persons with cancer or those being treated with anticancer drugs for tumors or other diseases, persons taking cortisone or prednisone or related drugs, generally should not be immunized.

Vaccines are usually grown in chicken or duck eggs so that if you have an allergy to eggs, alternate vaccination may be needed or desensitization should be accomplished before it is given.

what are the common vaccines?

The majority of common vaccines are given in early infancy and childhood according to a recognized schedule. These include diphtheria and tetanus toxoid and pertussis (whooping cough) vaccine which are usually combined as DPT. The vaccine for all three polio viruses is given orally (but should not be given when suffering from diarrhea). Measles, rubella and mumps virus vaccines are also preferably given in early childhood. Since diphtheria and pertussis are primarily childhood diseases, the only common vaccine which needs renewal in adulthood is tetanus toxoid, which should probably be renewed with a booster every 10 years. Further, if a person has a cut or wound associated with obviously dirty material such as rusty metal, there may be a need for passive immunization with tetanus antitoxin or tetanus immunoglobulin, depending on the number of previous tetanus immunizations and the type and age of the wound. The only other type of vaccinations necessary in adulthood, except those needed when travelling to areas where contagious diseases are endemic (see below), come when a person such as a hospital worker, is exposed to a disease, such as polio.

Several vaccines or antiserums are given in special circumstances. The requirements for the once-common smallpox vaccination are changing because of the almost complete elimination of this dread disease, although it sis still required for travel to a few countries, as is typhoid

influenza vaccines

vaccine. This is also true of plague, cholera, typhus or yellow fever vaccines.

The general recommendation for influenza vaccination is that the only persons who need it are those susceptible to severe effects from the illness, such as elderly persons or persons with severe lung disease such as emphysema, chronic bronchitis or with diabetes mellitus. This is because there is generally a high incidence of reactions (although usually mild, such as fever for several hours) and the immunity is variable and of short duration. Influenza viruses change in character frequently, necessitating new vaccine strains. One reason why the swine influenza vaccine was recommended in 1976 was that it was strongly felt that this particular influenza virus would be very likely to seriously affect younger people. But, in general, the previous practice of giving influenza vaccine to susceptible persons still applies.

The principle of preventive therapy in stimulating the body to create its own immunity is old, but continues to be a very promising area of medical research. In the future we may well see vaccines or other drugs which cause greater immunity for the hepatitis virus, the common cold and other common viruses. Immunotherapy is also being studied in treating cancer, but its usefulness it not yet known.

Drugs for skin and local disorders

Many external or local problems are highly visible, disfiguring and/or uncomfortable and a wide variety of preparations are made for application to the skin or body orifices, mostly to produce a local effect. There are literally hundreds of drugs used for local disorders, of which several rank among the most commonly prescribed medicines, and are described in Part III.

steroid
preparations

The most widely used topical (local) medications are the coricosteroid creams and ointments (see also Steroids or Cortisone-like Drugs) such as Valisone, Synalar, Cordran, Lidex, T.A.C. (triamcinolone) and hydrocortisone. These applications, which have a cortisone-like effect, are drugs of choice in many skin disorders with symptoms of inflammation and itching like eczema, neurodermatitis and psoriasis. Because of their rather dramatic effect on some skin ailments, indiscriminate use of these products on every skin lesion has led to occasional problems with longer-term use. Some of the corticosteroids applied to the skin are the same as those given orally or by injection, for example, hydrocortisone and triamcinolone. In a wide variety of steroids, fluorine has been added to the molecules to increase their strength and potency, as in Synalar and Valisone. After long use, these fluorinated steroids can produce shrinkage and other changes of the skin.

occlusive dressing

Topical corticosteroids seem to work better on moist skin, so moistening the skin is advisable before application. This has also led to development of the occlusive dressing. In conditions where steroids must be applied for many days, they are more effective if the area is covered with plastic wrap to seal in the moisture. This procedure is regularly used in psoriasis treatment. Long-term use of such topical corticosteroid creams often results in sufficient absorption of the drug to cause corticosteroid side effects and to decrease normal activity of the adrenal gland. The cost of many such Trade name preparations is very high, but equally effective preparations are available by generic name.

steroid plus antimicrobial drugs

A related group of locally applied drugs consists of steroid creams compounded with such antibiotic or antifungal drugs as Cortisporin, Mycolog, NeoDecadron and Vioform-Hydrocortisone. The rationale for this combination is the simultaneous attempt to reduce local inflammation and eliminate the infection. In some cases, this approach may be effective, but it is problematic which component has the effect, and in some cases, the steroid may prevent normal healing. The answer may be to use both, but separately and only as needed.

topical antibiotics

Topical antibiotics such as Neosporin and Bacitracin ointment find frequent use on small wounds and cuts. The effectiveness of these preparations has been questioned since it isn't clear whether the antibiotic in an ointment can really be active against skin bacteria, or is any better than simply keeping a wound clean and protected. Certain new topical preparations containing antibiotics such as tetracycline and erythromycin have been used in acne treatment and appear to be successful. Preparations containing the antibiotic neomycin (i.e. Neosporin, Cortispirin) have a fairly high incidence of skin sensitization, producing an allergic reaction.

antifungal preparations

As opposed to antibiotic creams and ointments, local antifungal preparations such as nystatin (Mycostatin), candicidin (Candeptin) and miconazole (Monistat) and Tinactin (tolnaftate) appear to be relatively effective applied locally. Because fungi are very persistent, the primary rule for treating fungus infections is to use a preparation regularly for the prescribed period, usually 10 days or more. Sensitization to these preparations is relatively low.

vaginal preparations

A specialized group of local antimicrobial preparations include creams or suppositories for vaginal infections. These occur most frequently in association with the use of birth control pills, but also through using antibiotics like tetracycline, or with diabetes. They may also occur without any obvious cause but are due to changes in the pH (acidity/alkalinity) and to the normal bacteria residing in the vagina. Under these conditions there is often a white discharge, with itching and burning. Vaginal discharge may be due to fungus infections, bacteria, Trichomonas or certain venereal disease like gonorrhea. The cause should be diagnosed by a physician or at a family planning clinic. If a fungal or Monilia infection is diagnosed, it is usually treated with antifungal creams like Mycostatin (mystatin), candicidin (Candeptin) or Monistat (miconazole). If it is due to Trichomonas, treatment will be with an oral drug, Flagyl, sometimes with treatment of the woman's partner if it is recurrent. If the problem is due to neither, it is probably a bacterial infection. In this case, and gonorrhea has been ruled out, vaginal creams containing sulfa drugs, such as AVC Cream, Sultrin Cream and Vagitrol, are frequently prescribed, although failure to use them for the prescribed course is a common mistake. Many gynecologists believe wearing cotton underwear and normalizing the acidity of the vagina with simple vinegar douching may eliminate the problem.

local anesthetics

An unrelated local problem is pain, as in cuts, sunburns and other minor superficial wounds. One of the most common treatments involves the use of drugs called local anesthetics. The Novocain, (procaine) and Xylocaine used by dentists to prevent pain are examples. Benzocaine is a common local anesthetic sold for relief of pain such as sunburn (Solarcaine). Many of these local anesthetics don't act on intact skin but may on burned skin or abrasions. The major concern about their use is the tendency for some local anesthetics, such as benzocaine, to cause allergic reactions. The general rule is to discontinue use if the condition worsens.

eye drops

There are a large number of medicines which are used directly on the eye. Most of these preparations act locally, on the pupil, cornea or lids, but they can sometimes be absorbed into the system and produce side effects. A variety of preparations are used. Antibiotics, in combination (as Neosporin eye drops), or alone, are often used for local infections or corneal scratches. Some corticosteroids are also used, with and without antibiotics. These are controversial, because although they are essential in preventing corneal scarring in some cases, they can worsen the condition when applied to virus lesions, as in Herpes of the eye. They can also predispose to fungal diseases of the eye if used for long periods.

Another common use of eye drops is for glaucoma. Glaucoma is a hereditary disorder which causes a block of normal fluid flow in the eye and can increase the pressure in the eye. This in turn can cause increased pressure on the retina and optic nerve and cause blindness. Local drugs, such as pilocarpine (Isopto Carpine) can relieve the pressure. Oral drugs, especially the diuretic Diamox, are also used to decrease this pressure.

Some factors are very important when medicines for the eye are considered. First, it is very important to keep the droppers sterile to prevent infections. Secondly, if different medicines are applied to each eye it is very important to have all of them marked to avoid confusion.

ear drops

The ear canal is a limited area where a few drugs are applied only to treat local infections or skin disorders. Since the eardrum closes the canal and forms a barrier, medicines do not usually reach the middle or inner ear by this route. If the eardrum is not intact, eardrops should generally be avoided. The most commonly used ear preparation is Cortisporin – a mixture of a steroid and antibiotics, discussed in Part III.

Listed below are some of the commonly prescribed drugs for skin and local disorders. Those marked with an asterisk are individually described in Part III.

Aristocort Derm.*	Kenalog Derm.*	TAC Cream
AVC Cream	Lidex*	Triple Sulfa
Cordran*	Mycolog*	Cream
Cortisporin	Mycostatin*	Valisone*
Flagyl*	Neosporin Eye	Vioform-
hydrocortisone	Drops*	Hydrocortisone*
cream	Sultrin Cream	
Isopto Carpine*	Synalar*	

Drugs for neurological disorders

Many neurological or neuromuscular disorders (that is, those that involve the brain and nerves and/or muscles) are due to gradual destruction of nerves or muscles from unknown causes. Multiple sclerosis and certain types of muscular dystrophy are examples. In other cases, such destruction is due to loss of blood supply to the brain as in a stroke. Medical science has not yet developed medicines that halt or reverse degenerative diseases, or reverse the effects of a stroke.

Thus, the use of medication in these diseases is limited to treating their symptoms such as muscle spasm, thought disorders or depression. There are some neurological disorders that do respond to drugs, the most common of these being migraine headaches (actually a disorder of the blood vessels to the brain), convulsions or seizures, and Parkinson's disease. These disorders are briefly discussed in the following sections.

Drugs for migraine

what brings on migraine?

True migraine headaches are often confused with other types of severe headaches, which are due to stress or tension. Tension also appears to precipitate true migraines in some people. Migraines are specific kinds of headaches, which may be preceded by a feeling (called an aura) that the headache is about to occur. Migraines often occur on one side of the head and may be accompanied by a loss of appetite, nausea and vomiting, and transitory visual changes. They may last for hours to days. Migraine headaches are associated with constriction of some of the arteries to the head (which may produce the aura), followed by relaxation of the arteries, which produces the severe pain. However, the reason this occurs is not known. Symptomatic treatment of mild migraine often involves the same analgesics or pain-relieving medicines used for other headaches, like aspirin or Darvon. But if the headache is severe, narcotics may be required to end the attack. Use of narcotics, even codeine, should be avoided because of the potential for addiction with recurrent use.

ergotamine: a valuable medicine to head off migraine

The most specific drug treatment for true vascular or migraine headaches, is ergotamine (Ergomar, Gynergen) taken at the first warning of an attack. It may be given by injection or taken by inhaling, dissolved under the tongue

105

or swallowed; with nausea or vomiting, the rectal suppository is effective. Ergotamine, which is derived from ergot, a fungus disease of rye plants, acts to constrict the arteries and possibly prevents the relaxation (pain) stage. Ergotamine is also combined with caffeine (in Cafergot) as well as with other drugs for sedation, nausea or to relieve pain (Cafergot P/B, Midrin, Bellergal, Wigraine, Migral). Caffeine appears to increase ergotamine absorption from the stomach, but the value of any such ingredients varies and has been questioned. Because there is a tendency for resistance, or tolerance to develop, regular use of ergotamine to prevent attacks may hinder effective treatment of an acute attack.

Sansert (methysergide) has been found to truly prevent recurrent attacks of migraine if taken regularly. However its use is usually discontinued at intervals due to serious side effects, which can result in extensive scar formation around the kidneys, lungs or heart. It is always used under careful medical supervision.

Listed below are some of the commonly prescribed drugs for migraine.

Bellergal   Caffergot   ergotamine

Drugs for seizures or convulsions

causes of
seizures

When certain parts of the brain are disturbed by injury, high fever, damage from a stroke or tumor, or from a congenital defect, there is the possibility that a seizure may occur. The seizure results from a brief disorganization of the brain's electrical impulses, which can be measured by an electroencephalograph (EEG). Physically, seizures range from localized twitches or arm movements, to rigidity of one side, or of the entire body (grand mal seizure), or by a sudden fall to the floor (akinetic seizures). The most common type of seizure has no known external cause, and is called idiopathic epilepsy. The majority of persons with seizure disorders can, with proper treatment, function quite normally.

There are only a few drugs suitable for treating epilepsy, and they are geared to the type of seizure being prevented. Only in rare cases, where seizures persist, must the seizure itself be treated with intravenous drugs such as Valium or Amobarbital.

The drugs used to treat epilepsy include drugs from three chemical groups: the barbiturates, such as phenobarbital, methylbarbital (Mebaral), primidone (Mysoline); the hydantoins, Dilantin (phenytoin), mephenytoin (Mesantoin); and the succinimides, Zarontin, Celontin and Milontin.

dilantin and phenobarbital: the major anticonvulsants

By far the most commonly used anticonvulsant drugs are Dilantin and phenobarbital. Treatment for epilepsy is often started with one of these two anticonvulsant drugs, and the dose adjusted to prevent seizures. If one drug in normal dosage is not effective alone, the other may be taken at the same time, depending on the type of seizure. Although childhood idiopathic seizures do not require life-long therapy, those occurring in adulthood, such as after head injury, may. This requires initial physical and psychological adjustment to therapy, but once stability has been achieved, should represent no major problem. Long-term use of both drugs mentioned can lead to adverse effects which are discussed in Part III. In most cases, the drugs are well tolerated, but if they are stopped suddenly, especially phenobarbital, a seizure called status epilepticus (a series of fits in unconsciousness) may occur, requiring diazepam administered intravenously.

Listed below are some of the commonly prescribed drugs for seizures or convulsions. Those with an asterisk are individually described in Part III.

Clonazepan	Mesantoin	Valium*
Dilantin*	phenobarbital*	
Mebaral	primidone	

Drugs for Parkinson's disease

characteristic Parkinsonian symptoms

Parkinson's disease is a brain disorder with a characteristic set of symptoms, all or some of which may be present. These symptoms include tremor of the hands, feet and sometimes the head, which is greater at rest; rigidity of the arms and legs; slowness of movement; loss of facial expression, a tendency to drool; and mental deterioration. Often these symptoms may be very mild and progress very slowly. This set of symptoms may be seen not only with Parkinson's disease but also commonly as a side effect of therapy with major tranquilizers such as Thorazine.

role of dopamine in the brain

The symptoms seem to be due to damage or degeneration of a very specific part of the brain. In cases not related to drugs, Parkinsonism is due to deficiency of a substance in the brain called dopamine. This substance and another, called acetylcholine, balance each other, making body movement smooth and coordinated. When there is not enough dopamine, acetylcholine is assumed to cause the symptoms. These facts form the basis for drug therapy in Parkinson's disease: medication to either increase dopamine levels, or block the effects of acetycholine.

Until the last few years, only one group of drugs was available, the acetylcholine blocking or anticholinergic drugs, the most commonly used being Artane (trihexyphenidyl) and Cogentin (benztropine). These are prescribed for types of Parkinson's symptoms and are the only drugs effective in cases due to major tranquilizer usage. They are used to treat mild Parkinsonism, though their effect tends to grow weaker with continued use.

levodopa: almost an answer

Treatment of Parkinson's disease was changed considerably several years ago with the introduction of levodopa (Dopar) which is converted into dopamine by the body. Initially hailed as the therapeutic answer to Parkinson's disease, levodopa's side effects have caused it to be reserved for more difficult cases. Nonetheless, it has considerably widened the possibilities of treatment, allowing many persons to function normally, despite some side effects, for much longer. A refinement to levodopa therapy was addition of carbidopa in a combination product (Sinemet), which decreases side effects.

A third useful drug was introduced as an antiviral agent called amantadine (Symmetrel). It is now used alone in mild cases of Parkindon's disease, or in combinations of the other two types of drugs, although it is only effective in some cases.

mild cases

Treatment of mild cases frequently is initiated with an anticholinergic drug (for example, Artane or Cogentin) or amantadine, often in conjunction with therapy aimed at exercising muscle function, and decreasing stress or tension. Levodopa or Sinemet is later added or substituted after gradual withdrawal of other drugs.

There is still much to be desired in improving the therapy of Parkinson's disease, particularly with respect to the frequency that the drugs must be taken, and their side effects. But the fact that drugs can correct very minute biochemical abnormalities in the brain brings some hope for development of more specific medication for this and related disorders in the future.

Listed below are some of the commonly prescribed drugs for Parkinson's disease. Those with an asterisk are individually described in Part III.

Artane*   Cogentin   L-dopa.

Drugs for gout

how gout begins: the painful crystals

Gout is an arthritis-like disease that can cause very painful, red and swollen joints, often first in the big toe during an acute attack. Chronic gout can cause degeneration of joints, in addition to formation of characteristic crystalline deposits of uric acid salts, called tophi, around the joints and cartilage and in the kidney. Gout is caused by an excess of uric acid in the blood. There appears to be a genetic predisposition to gout, although it can arise in association with certain blood diseases, tumors, or cancer therapy. Men are more likely than women to have this form of arthritis.

Uric acid is formed from the breakdown of nucleic acids (DNA and RNA) which are present in every cell in the body. In addition, a small quantity of uric acid is derived from the diet, especially from such foods as brain, heart, liver and sweetbreads and certain seafood, including anchovy, lobster and sardines. Some people with gout are therefore advised to avoid such foods. Alcohol, particularly in excess, may also increase uric acid levels. These facts lent partial credence to the notion that gout was an affliction of the rich, brought on by rich foods and large quantities of wine.

treating an attack

Drugs for gout are used to treat an acute attack and to prevent recurrent attacks. These include colchicine, oxyphenbutazone (Tandearil), phenylbutazone (Butazolidin), and rarely, indomethacin (Indocin). These medications reduce inflammation, but have little effect on the primary disease. Colchicine is quite specific for acute attacks of gout, providing striking relief, and diagnostic proof, in an authentic attack. As detailed below, colchicine is sometimes taken in small doses with drugs to prevent

preventing attacks

recurrent attacks. Medication taken to prevent recurrent attacks act to decrease the amount of uric acid in the body. Two commonly used older drugs, probenecid (Benemid) and sulfinpyrazone (Anturane), promote elimination of uric acid by the kidneys. (Probenecid is also available combined with colchincine as Colbenemid. Allopurinol (Zyloprim), often more effective than the older drugs, acts by inhibiting an enzyme that is essential to the breakdown of body cell constituents into uric acid.

When treatment is started with any of the three preventive drugs, there is a risk that an acute attack of gout may occur. Consequently, colchicine or another anti-inflammatory drug is also given for a few weeks.

precautions during gout therapy

Although diet restrictions are no longer necessary when taking anti-gout medication, many diuretics (see Diuretics) tend to raise uric acid levels by reducing its elimination by the kidneys. These small increases do not usually cause gout, but it is necessary to measure the blood level of uric acid at intervals and sometimes to discontinue the diuretic. Aspirin and other salicylates should not be taken in large doses or continually with most drugs used for gout (although this does not apply to allupurinol), but acetaminophen can be taken if an analgesic is required. In order to avoid kidney damage, or the possibility of stone formation, plenty of liquids should be drunk – about three quarts daily.

Listed below are some of the commonly prescribed drugs for gout. Those with an asterisk are individually described in Part III.

Anturane   Colbenemid   Zyloprim*
Benemid   colchicine

Vitamins and minerals

Vitamins and minerals are nutrient substances essential for human body growth and function. The amounts required are often very tiny when compared to the amounts often sold and taken by the American public.

There is much confusion in the subject of vitamins and minerals, as well as other substances termed "nutritional supplements" such as lecithin, kelp, garlic, and so on. There is a vast amount of material written on the subject – some in scientific journals, but the majority in the form of personal testimonials about the value of particular vitamins or specially formulated mixtures of these substances. The whole controversial issue cannot be addressed but a few useful facts may be presented.

are vitamins and minerals drugs?

Most experts do not view vitamins and minerals as drugs, yet in many respects they have some similarities to drugs and hormones. For example, vitamins travel essentially the same route as drugs from the stomach to the liver to the bloodstream, to their place of action, and finally to the kidney, where they are eliminated. When taken in high doses (especially fat soluble vitamins), they can cause ill-effects, and they do interact with medicines. Like drugs, they affect many tissues and organs, and in the case of some vitamins, we are just now beginning to understand their important actions. (Vitamin D is felt by some to be more properly called a hormone, since it is produced in the body after exposure to the sun and has some resemblance to cortisone; however, it is not produced by a gland, which would distinguish it from other hormones.)

The normal varied diet of an adult usually contains most of the required vitamins and minerals in adequate amounts. It has never been shown that a healthy person on a well-rounded diet benefits in any way from vitamin or mineral supplements. In fact, rarely is the average person who feels "run down" or "tired" actually suffering from a lack of vitamins or minerals, especially if a normal diet has been followed.

are vitamins really useful?

Despite the fact that a normal diet eliminates the need for vitamin and mineral supplements in most cases, there are situations where additional vitamins may be essential. However, it should be noted that many foods such as milk, margarine and bread *are* supplemented with vitamins so that again, requirements may often be met through diet, rather than taking pills. Recent food labeling laws require listing vitamins and minerals, which allows calculation of intake.

Those situations where vitamins and minerals *are* needed include conditions where there is an increased demand for vitamins, such as during growth, in infancy and childhood, and during pregnancy and lactation. Occasionally this applies in prolonged, severe illnesses, especially where there has been fever. A decreased vitamin supply can be due to a poor diet either from excess consumption of carbohydrate and fat and few vegetables, or from certain fad diets. A decreased supply to the body can result if vitamins are not absorbed due to chronic diarrhea or diseases causing malabsorption. Supplies of vitamins and minerals can be exhausted, but once replenished and a normal diet is resumed, supplements are not always necessary.

Some vitamins and minerals are essentially used as

drugs. For example, vitamin C (ascorbic acid) has the ability to make the urine acid. It is sometimes used in this way, often in relatively large doses, to acidify the urine and help prevent urinary infections (bacteria do not grow well in acid urine). The mineral calcium in the form of a salt (calcium carbonate) is used in some antacids to neutralize stomach acid. Finally, the mineral potassium chloride is often taken to replace the potassium lost when a diuretic is given.

There are some basic differences between the two major types of vitamins (fat soluble and water soluble) as well as minerals.

fat soluble vitamins

The fat soluble vitamins, A,D,E and K are so-called because they are more soluble in fat than in water, and their absorption from the intestines is similar to the absorption of fat. These vitamins are stored in the liver and eliminated very slowly, so that excessive doses can accumulate and cause serious problems and illness (especially vitamins A and D). Deficiences of these vitamins may occur when there is poor absorption in the intestine (malabsorption, chronic diarrhea or excessive use of laxatives). These vitamins are measured in units of activity called international units (I.U.). In general, an I.U. represents a specific amount of biological activity in a biological test system.

water soluble vitamins

The water soluble vitamins, which include vitamin C (ascorbic acid), the B complex (B1-thiamine, B2-riboflavin, B6-pyridoxine, B12-cyanocobalamin), niacin, folic acid, pantothenic acid and biotin are found in many plants and animals. They act at sites throughout the body and are rapidly eliminated in the urine. Accumulation is unlikely with normal kidneys, and adverse effects of excessive doses, with the exception of niacin, are not common. Amounts of these vitamins are usually expressed in terms of weight in milligrams.

minerals

Minerals are simple elemental substances which occur as organic and inorganic complexes or "salts" that are necessary to the makeup of all tissues and fluids. Common table salt (sodium chloride) is the most well-known and essential mineral; it is present both inside and outside of all living cells. Minerals are sometimes classified as *macro-*minerals and *trace* minerals. The minerals calcium, sodium, potassium, magnesium, phosphorus, sulphur and chlorine are present in the body in relatively large amounts and occur in most cells. They are often referred to as the *macro*-minerals and requirements are expressed in milligrams. The *trace* minerals such as zinc, iron, iodine, copper, cobalt, chromium, fluorine and manganese, among others, are present in much smaller amounts and are often complexed with proteins to affect their structure or function (as in enzymes). The amounts usually required are much smaller and less is known about the actual function and essential nature of many, such as manganese and zinc. However, iodine and iron are well understood and their function is known to be quite essential.

how mush is needed?

The Food and Nutrition Board of the National Research Council has studied the available data and established "Recommended Daily Allowances" (RDA) for dietary supplements. This is *different* than the United States Recommended Daily Allowances (USRDA) which is a set of values for *labeling* purposes. The RDA allowances have been established as amounts necessary to maintain good nutrition in most healthy persons. They have been established for various age groups and for pregnant and lactating women.

It is important to understand that if certain vitamins are taken in excess, they may create relative deficiencies of other nutrients. For example, B-complex vitamins often occur together in nature and are best taken in balanced amounts, except in special cases where only one is known to be depleted. It is partly for this reason, plus the fact that vitamin and mineral deficiencies are more often multiple than isolated, that some multivitamin preparations are sensible in treatment of general nutritional deficiency. It is currently thought by some authorities that an appropriate multivitamin should contain only the substances and amounts proportional to those established by the RDA. Those containing other substances such as choline, bioflavonoids or inositol are of unknown value.

dietary supplements

It is very important to note that there are at least four different types of multivitamin preparations, each of which has different uses. First are the dietary supplements or prophylactic vitamins, which contain no more than one to one and a half times the RDA, and may be useful in preventing mild deficiencies during dieting or short illnesses.

therapeutic multivitamins

The second type are the therapeutic multivitamins, which may contain three to five times the RDA – except for vitamins A, D and folic acid. Excess A and D can cause poisoning, while excess folic acid can mask pernicious anemia. The usual use for these is in true nutritional deficiency associated with alcoholism, malabsorption or gastrointestinal surgery. Their use for any length of time should be supervised by a physician.

vitamins for pregnancy and lactation

A third type of multivitamins are those which have been formulated to the requirements of pregnant and lactating women, but their composition varies considerably from brand to brand. In general, those containing more than five times the RDA of any ingredient, more than 10,000 I.U.s of vitamin A or 4,000 units of vitamin D are not as appropriate as a combination containing recommended amounts.

vitamins with minerals

The fourth category of multivitamins are those which also contain mineral supplements. Except for calcium, iron and possibly fluoride, the specific needs and usefulness of the added minerals is not very well known. Calcium may be useful in pregnancy and lactation, iron in conditions where there is blood loss (most commonly in women with heavy menstrual periods; healthy men who have no bleeding problems almost never need iron), and fluoride when the local water is deficient. Much is being written about the value of the other trace minerals, but generally they are obtained in very adequate amounts in the diet.

cost

Vitamin preparations vary considerably in cost and higher cost does not necessarily assure greater benefit. With the RDA requirements kept in mind, a generic multivitamin at lower cost may be found to be essentially equivalent to high-priced preparations. In most cases, a good varied diet should eliminate the need for the expenditure entirely, except in true deficiency.

Listed below are some of the commonly prescribed vitamins and minerals. Those with an asterisk are individually described in Part III.

Feosol*	potassium	Tri-Vi-Flor Drops*
Poly Vi-Flor	chloride*	
Chewable*	Slow-K*	

Part III An Alphabetical Guide to Over 200 of the Most Frequently Prescribed Drugs

Acetaminophen

trade names

> Tylenol, Nebs, Tempra, Datril

action and uses
A popular mild pain reliever used as an alternative to aspirin. Like aspirin, it can also reduce fever. Unlike aspirin, it has no anti-inflammatory effects, but it also has fewer side effects and drug interactions. It is present in a large number of pain relieving combination drugs. Another common pain reliever, phenacetin, is actually converted to acetaminophen in the body.

adult dosage
Two 325 mg tablets every 4-6 hours as needed for pain or fever.

adverse effects
In usual doses, there are few adverse effects, although excessive doses can cause liver damage. As opposed to the similar phenacetin, this drug does not cause kidney damage.

precautions
Excessive doses over long periods may cause liver damage. This very popular drug is a very common cause of accidental and often *untreatable* overdosage in children. It should always be kept well out of their reach.

drug interactions
Rarely, this drug may increase the effects of anticoagulants or major tranquilizers, but this is of questionable significance.

see essay
Non-Narcotic Pain Relievers.

Acetazolamide (generic name). See DIAMOX ORAL.

Achromycin-V

generic name

> tetracycline (available by generic name)

115

action and uses
One of the most commonly used oral antibiotics. In the generic form it was the 4th most frequently prescribed drug in 1976. There are a number of tetracycline drugs available, but most are comparable in their actions and side effects except for Minocin and Vibramycin. Achromycin-V (tetracycline) is known as a "broad spectrum" antibiotic because it can be used in a wide variety of different infections, although it is the first choice drug in very few common infections. It acts by stopping the production of proteins in sensitive bacterial cells with little effect on human cells. Tetracycline is currently very commonly used in low doses to inhibit the bacteria on the face which are believed to contribute to acne. It is also frequently used by those with chronic bronchitis or other lung disease. Less frequently it is used to treat urinary tract infections or venereal disease when penicillin allergy is present. It has no effect on viral illnesses, including colds, or on fungus infections.

adult dosage
The usual oral dose is 250 or 500 mg every six hours for a prescribed number of days as specified by the physician. It is very important to take this on an empty stomach. The dose may vary in some cases such as acne, where it may be lower.

adverse effects
Achromycin-V commonly can cause various gastrointestinal symptoms including nausea and vomiting, burning stomach or belching, cramps and diarrhea. The latter symptom is often due to the fact that tetracycline inhibits some bacteria in the lower intestine and elsewhere and allows overgrowth of other bacteria (normally held in check) and minor fungi. This can also result in vaginal infection, anorectal itching and a sore mouth (thrush). These symptoms tend to disappear when the drug is discontinued. Less commonly, tetracycline can cause rashes, or other allergic reactions and sensitivity of the skin to sunlight causing rashes (photosensitivity). It can also tend to worsen certain types of kidney disease, and rarely cause liver damage or blood cell abnormalities.

precautions
Tetracycline should not be taken by pregnant or potentially pregnant or nursing women, and should be used with caution when significant liver or kidney disease is present. This antibiotic, like all others, should be taken for the time period directed, and every dose should be taken. Failure to do this can result in inadequate treatment of the infection, recurrence or development of resistant infections.

drug interactions
The most common drug interaction is between tetracyc-

line and antacids or milk products, since the tetracycline binds to these and does not get into the body. Tetracycline can potentially increase the effect of the anticoagulant Coumadin and increase the hazard of bleeding.

see essay
Drugs to Treat Infections.

Actifed

generic
ingredients

> antihistamine = tripolidine hydrochloride
> decongestant = pseudoephedrine hydrochloride

Actifed C Expectorant

generic
ingredients

> antihistamine = tripolidine hydrochloride
> decongestant = pseudoephedrine hydrochloride
> narcotic = codeine phosphate
> expectorant = glyceryl guaiacolate

action and uses
Actifed is a combination drug used to control seasonal or perennial allergic rhinitis (runny nose) which may be due to specific irritants, such as the pollen of trees or grass, or may even be caused by emotional stress or worry, grief or other upsetting experiences (vasomotor rhinitis). The decongestant part of Actifed shrinks the linings of the nose and respiratory passages. The antihistamine blocks the substance (histamine) which causes the breathing passages to swell and discharge mucus. In addition to these ingredients, Actifed C Expectorant contains codeine phosphate, used here not as a painkiller but to control cough, and the expectorant glyceryl guaiacolate, which helps to liquefy the mucus blocking up the breathing passages. These effects might counteract each other. Actifed C provides cough-suppressant, expectorant, decongestant and antihistamine effects.

adult dosage
Actifed: 1 tablet 3 times a day or 2 teaspoonfuls of the syrup 3 times a day. Actifed C Expectorant: the usual dose is 2 teaspoonfuls (10 ml) 4 times per day. For severe cases the above dosages may be reduced by half and given every 3 hours.

adverse effects
Side effects may include drowsiness due to the antihistamine and possibly palpitation due to the decongestants. Although the amount of codeine is small, it may cause nausea and vomiting, and if used for several days, may cause constipation. The expectorant may cause nausea.

precautions This drug should be avoided by pregnant, potentially pregnant and nursing women. Driving or operating heavy equipment may be hazardous if sedation is an effect of this medication. Persons taking medicine for high blood pressure or heart ailments should check with their physicians before using, since the decongestants may elevate the blood pressure. Repeated use for any period of more than 2-4 days should be avoided in most cases.

drug dependence The codeine in this compound can cause habituation if taken for prolonged periods.

drug interactions The sedative effects of the antihistamine, and to a lesser extent the codeine, can be additive to any other sedating drug such as tranquilizers and alcohol. The decongestants can raise the blood pressure and thus counteract the effect of any drug used to treat high blood pressure. Like most drugs of this type, Actifed may add to the effects of antispasmodic drugs used for stomach disorders, such as Pro-Banthine and Librax. This can cause excessive mouth dryness and difficulty in urinating.

see essay *Drugs for Coughs and Colds.*

Afrin

generic name

oxymetazoline hydrochloride

action and uses A nasal decongestant used to relieve congestion of the nose, sinuses and throat. Afrin decreases the flow of blood to the tissues lining the nasal passages, the sinuses and the throat, and thereby relieves congestion. It is used to counter the symptoms of a variety of allergies and infections including the common cold. After prolonged use Afrin may lose its effectiveness.

adult dosage Usually 2 or 3 squeezes of the nasal spray in each nostril, twice a day. Afrin also comes as a liquid with a dropper. The usual dosage is one dropper-full in each nostril not more than twice a day.

adverse effects Side effects include burning, stinging and dryness of the nasal passages. Some individuals may experience nervousness, headache, lightheadedness and sleeplessness, and some may suffer from pounding of the heart (palpitations) and elevation of the blood pressure.

precautions Afrin should be avoided in persons who have heart disease or high blood pressure or are taking medicines for these conditions.

drug interactions — Afrin can cause elevation of the blood pressure and other reactions in persons taking drugs for depression (MAO inhibitors or tricyclic antidepressants) or for high blood pressure, such as reserpine.

see essay — *Drugs for Coughs and Colds.*

Aldactazide

generic ingredients

> diuretics=spironolactone
> =hydrochlorothiazide

action and uses — A fixed-dose combination of two diuretics ("water pills") used in the treatment disorders that cause excessive retention of salt and water and high blood pressure. One component is spironolactone, a drug which, by blocking the hormone aldosterone, causes the body to eliminate excess water and salt, but not potassium. (This essential mineral tends to be eliminated along with salt and water in the case of most other diuretics). The second, somewhat stronger, diuretic is hydrochlorothiazide. Although the diuretic effects of its two ingredients are additive, Aldactazide, like other fixed-dose combinations, has several disadvantages: the dosage of one component cannot be adjusted without affecting the dosage of the other; it has an increased number of side effects; and it is more expensive than other, equally effective products.

adult dosage — Usually 2–4 tablets per day in divided doses. (Each tablet of Aldactazide contains 25 mg of spironolactone and 25 mg of hydrochlorothiazide).

adverse effects — Possible side effects with spironolactone can include the retention of waste products by the kidney, headache, drowsiness, skin rash, breast enlargement, and irregular menstrual periods. Possible side effects with hydrochlorothiazide include a rise in the body's blood sugar level, which can precipitate diabetes, and a rise in the body's uric acid level, which can precipitate gout. Both drugs can cause allergic reactions.

precautions — Aldactazide should not be used by pregnant or potentially pregnant women, and by patients with kidney disorders.

drug interactions — Because of the spironolactone in Aldactazide, a dangerous rise in the body's potassium level is possible if supplementary potassium (KCl or Slow-K) is taken concurrently.

see essays — *Drugs for High Blood Pressure. Diuretics.*

119

Aldactone

generic name

> spironolactone

action and uses
A mild diuretic ("water pill") used to treat the excessive water retention caused by certain heart, liver and kidney diseases and by some types of high blood pressure. A major part of these disorders tends to be the overproduction of aldosterone, a hormone which encourages the body to retain its salt and water and eliminate the mineral potassium. Aldactone works by blocking this hormone – thus making it possible for the body to eliminate excess salt and water and retain potassium. (Most other diuretics do not prevent the loss of this essential mineral. However, although this effect may be advantageous when there is a need to prevent excess potassium loss, the advantage must be weighed against the problems and expense of using Aldactone).

adult dosage
Usually 50-300 mg per day, divided into several doses. Often Aldactone's effect will not be felt until the effects of the hormone aldosterone have worn off – which can take as long as three days.

adverse effects
Aldactone has a high incidence of side effects. Paradoxically, the major adverse effect is a dangerous, even life-threatening, increase in the body's potassium level, particularly if supplementary potassium is being taken (a common practice when other, stronger diuretics are also in use). For this reason, blood tests should be made at intervals to check the body's potassium level. Another side effect that should be checked by occasional blood tests is a decrease in the kidney's ability to eliminate waste products. Other side effects may include headache, drowsiness, skin rash, breast enlargement and irregular menstrual periods.

precautions
Aldactone should not be used by pregnant or potentially pregnant women and should be used with caution by patients with a kidney disorder.

drug interactions
Hazardous high potassium levels are possible if Aldactone is taken along with supplementary potassium such as Slow-K or KCl.

see essays
Drugs for High Blood Pressure. Diuretics.

Aldomet

generic name

> methyldopa

action and uses

A drug used to treat high blood pressure. It works by blocking the sympathetic nervous system to cause relaxation of the walls of the blood vessels. Usually prescribed with a diuretic ("water pill") to enhance its effect. Aldomet is, in fact, often the second drug tried when a diuretic alone has not succeeded in lowering the blood pressure.

adult dosage

The usual daily dose is 500 mg 2-4 times per day. Initially, the dose may be 250 mg 2-3 times per day, with a dosage adjustment at intervals until the desired effect is produced or a daily total of 2 grams is reached.

adverse effects

Initially, most patients experience drowsiness or lethargy, but these effects usually wear off within two to three weeks. Less common side effects may include dry mouth, stuffy nose, lightheadedness on moving suddenly, skin rash, depression, nightmares, joint and muscle pain, nausea, and changes in sexual function. Some of these effects may decrease with time. More rarely, abnormalities of blood cells or the liver may occur.

precautions

Because Aldomet can cause marked drowsiness when first started, driving and operating heavy equipment should be avoided. The drug should be avoided if possible in pregnant, potentially pregnant or nursing women.

drug interactions

Aldomet can interact with many other drugs, and the doctor's advice should be sought after before taking *any* other prescription or over-the-counter drug. Drugs that can seriously impair Aldomet's effectiveness and lead to a rise in blood pressure include antidepressants like Elavil, Tofranil and Sinequan; major tranquilizers like Thorazine; MAO inhibitor drugs like Nardil; amphetamines like Dexedrine and Benzedrine; appetite suppressants like Preludin; nasal sprays like Neosynephrine; and decongestant cough, cold, asthma and allergy drugs like Actifed.

see essays

Drugs for High Blood Pressure. Diuretics.

Aldoril

generic
ingredients

> diuretic=hydrochlorothiazide
> antihypertensive = methyldopa

action and uses One of several popular fixed combination drugs used to treat high blood pressure. Aldoril contains two types of antihypertensive drug: methyldopa, which acts on the sympathetic nervous system to relax the walls of the blood vessels, and hydrochlorothiazide, a diuretic which causes the kidneys to eliminate salt and water, thus reducing the amount of fluid in the blood and body tissues. Like other fixed combination drugs, Aldoril has several disadvantages: its dosage is inflexible (the amount of one ingredient cannot be altered without affecting the amount of the other); it increases the number of side effects; and it is more expensive than equally effective single-ingredient products.

adult dosage Usually 2-6 tablets per day in divided doses. The drug comes in two strengths: Aldoril-15, which contains 15 mg of hydrochlorothiazide and 250 mg of methyldopa; and Aldoril-25, which contains 25 mg of hydrochlorothiazide and 250 mg of methyldopa.

adverse effects The hydrochlorothiazide in Aldoril may cause an excessive loss of the mineral potassium, which may result in dizziness, unusual tiredness, muscle cramps and or tingling in the extremities. Fortunately, it is easy to replace lost potassium by adding high-potassium foods, such as dried fruits and bananas, citrus fruits and tomato juice to the diet; by using salt substitutes such as Lite-Salt; or with a supplement of potassium chloride liquid (KCl). The amount of loss and the need for potassium replacement can be ascertained by regular blood tests. Other side effects from hydrochlorothiazide may include an elevation of the blood sugar level in patients predisposed to diabetes, and a rise in the body's uric acid level which may predispose to gout. Both these effects can be watched for, and rarely produce problems. Finally, some people are allergic to hydrochlorothiazide and develop reactive skin rashes.

The methyldopa in Aldoril may cause drowsiness or lethargy, dry mouth and nasal stuffiness, and lightheadedness on changing position suddenly, but these effects tend to disappear in 2 to 4 weeks. Less frequently, the methlydopa in Aldoril can cause skin rash, nausea, depression, nightmares, joint and muscle pain, liver or blood abnormalities, and changes in sexual function.

precautions Because Aldoril can cause marked drowsiness when first started, driving and operating heavy equipment should be avoided. It should be avoided if possible by pregnant, potentially pregnant or nursing women. The blood potassium level should be checked or potassium taken if digoxin is also being taken.

drug interactions   Cortisone and cortisone-like drugs such as prednisone can interact with the hydrochlorothiazide in Aldoril to cause excessive potassium loss. Potentially serious interactions may also occur with digitalis drugs for the heart because if and when too much potassium is eliminated from the system by the hydrochlorothiazide, the heart becomes sensitive to the toxic effects of digitalis. Drugs that may impair the blood pressure-lowering effect of the methyldopa in Aldoril include antidepressants like Elavil, Tofranil and Sinequan; major tranquilizers like Thorazine; MAO inhibitor drugs like Nardil; amphetamines like Dexedrine and Benzedrine; appetite suppressants like Preludin; nasal sprays like Neosynephrine; and decongestant drugs for coughs, colds, asthma or allergies, like Actifed. Finally, alcohol, barbiturates, sedatives and pain relievers may be additive to Aldoril's sedative effect. The doctor should be consulted before any prescription or over-the-counter drug is taken while a patient is on Aldoril.

see essays   *Drugs for High Blood Pressure. Diuretics.*

Ambenyl Expectorant

generic
ingredients

antihistamines =	diphenhydramine
=	bromodiphenhydramine
expectorants =	ammonium chloride
=	guaiacolsulfonate
miscellaneous =	chloroform
=	menthol
=	alcohol
narcotic cough suppressant =	codeine

action and uses   A widely prescribed cough mixture containing two antihistamines which are also believed to have a mild cough suppressant effect, and expectorants, which are believed to help liquify bronchial secretions. In fact, the effectiveness of this and other similar cough syrups is difficult to establish. The inclusion of codeine makes this mixture restricted for use, since it suppresses coughing, which is often desirable.

adult dosage   Usually two teaspoonfuls every 4 hours, not to exceed 12 teaspoons per 24 hours.

adverse effects   The antihistamine can cause drowsiness, and less frequently, dizziness. The expectorants can sometimes cause nausea. The codeine, although present in small amounts,

123

may also cause nausea and constipation.

precautions

If drowsiness occurs, it may interfere with driving and operating machinery. Ambenyl should be avoided by pregnant or potentially pregnant women or nursing mothers.

drug
dependence

The codeine, if taken for prolonged periods in excessive doses, can potentially result in habituation.

drug interactions

The antihistamine and codeine in Ambenyl can add to the effects of alcohol, tranquilizers and sleeping pills, as well as antispasmodic anticholinergic drugs such as Pro-Banthine or Librax. Because of the alcohol, Benylin can cause a hazardous interaction if Flagyl or Antabuse is also taken.

see essays

Drugs for Coughs and Colds. Antihistamines.

Amcill

generic name

ampicillin (available by generic name)

Amcill is a trade name for ampicillin and is described fully under that heading below.

Amoxil

generic name

amoxicillin

action and uses

Amoxil is almost identical to ampicillin in its actions, uses and side effects except that it can be taken without regard to meals, while ampicillin must be taken on an empty stomach. See the detailed discussion on ampicillin below.

Amoxicillin (generic name). See AMOXIL, LAROTID.

Ampicillin

trade names

Amcill, Omnipen, Pen-A, Penbritin, Pensyn, Polycillin, Principen, Supen, Alpen, Totacillin

actions and uses

An antibiotic used to treat many infections including those of the urinary tract, ear, nose and throat. It is one of several so-called "semi-synthetic" penicillins which is made by both chemical and biological manipulations of penicillin produced by the mold *penicillium*.

Ampicillin, like penicillin, acts by preventing bacteria

from forming their cell walls. They therefore break up. It has no effect on human cells since they have a different structure. Though basic penicillin G is still one of the most important of all the antibiotics, it has several disadvantages. One is its somewhat limited effectiveness against the gram negative organisms. Another disadvantage is that it is not totally effective when taken by mouth because penicillin G is broken down by stomach acid. Ampicillin is highly effective when given by mouth on an empty stomach because it is not broken down by stomach acids. Because it is active against many kinds of bacteria, it is called a "broad spectrum" antibiotic. It is less effective than penicillin G against Gram positive cocci (found in abcesses and ear infections), but more effective against Gram negative bacteria which cause urinary tract infections. It is not effective against fungus or virus diseases. Antibiotics should not be used for trivial infections or to treat non-sensitive bacteria; such use only produces resistant bacteria which are difficult to eliminate.

adult dosage

The average adult dose is 250 mg or 500 mg every 6 hours on an empty stomach or at least 2 hours after a meal. The dosage should always be advised by a physician and will vary with the type and severity of infection.

adverse effects

Many people develop allergic reactions to the penicillin group of drugs. Once sensitization develops, *all* forms of penicillin including ampicillin can produce a reaction. An allergic reaction is characterized by either skin rashes, hives, itching, fever, difficulty in breathing, or swelling of the lips and tongue. Persons who have infectious mononucleosis often develop rashes due to ampicillin and should not take it while they have the disease. Ampicillin can also produce stomach upset due to the killing of certain normal bacteria in the intestine, and may cause diarrhea. It may also cause mild fungus infections of the anorectal area or vagina.

precautions

This antibiotic should not be used if there is a history of allergy to any type of penicillin. Due to a high frequency of rashes, it should not be taken by persons with infectious mononucleosis. Once a course of ampicillin is begun, it should be taken for its entire course of not less than 5-7 days, unless of course, side effects occur. It should not be stopped when the infections seems to be gone, since the infection can recur. The frequent starting and stopping of any antibiotic only leads to the development of resistant bacteria which are much more difficult to treat. Nursing mothers should ask the physician's advice.

drug interactions The effectiveness of ampicillin may be hindered by the antibiotics erythromycin and chloramphenicol, if they are used together. Food and antacids may interfere with the absorption of this drug.

see essay *Drugs to Treat Infections.*

Antivert

generic name

meclizine (available by generic name)

action and uses An antihistamine prescribed for the control of the nausea, vomiting and dizziness associated with motion sickness. It is also used to treat Meniere's syndrome and other disorders that affect the center of equilibrium in the inner ear and produce vertigo (the sensation that one's surroundings are spinning). It has the other actions of antihistamines and is sometimes used for allergies or itching.

adult dosage For the prevention of motion sickness, the usual dose is 25 – 50 mg one hour before embarkation. The dose may be repeated every 6 – 8 hours for the duration of the journey as needed. For the control of the dizziness caused by disorders affecting the inner ear, the usual dose is 25 – 100 mg per day in divided doses. It is advisable to begin with a low dose and adjust as needed until the dizziness is controlled or a maximum of 100 mg per day is reached. This drug may also be purchased without a prescription.

adverse effects Antivert may cause drowsiness, blurred vision, or dryness of the nose, mouth or throat. Rashes may rarely occur.

precautions It must not be used during pregnancy because tests have shown that it causes birth defects in animals. It should be used with caution by those planning to drive a car or operate heavy machinery while under the effects of the drug.

drug interactions Oversedation may result if Antivert is taken in combination with alcohol, sleeping pills, tranquilizers, antidepressants, pain relievers, drugs containing narcotics, and other antihistamines.

see essays *Antihistamines. Drugs for Nausea, Stomach Upset and Ulcers.*

Apresoline

generic name

> hydralazine (available by generic name)

action and uses

A drug used to lower blood pressure by relaxing, and therefore dilating, arterial blood vessels. It is used in treating mild to moderate hypertension, and is usually used in conjunction with a diuretic ("water pill") and or a drug that prevents the sympathetic nervous system from constricting the blood vessels, such as Aldomet, or reserpine.

adult dosage

As response to this drug varies considerably, it is usually started at a dose of 10 mg 3-4 times per day and gradually increased, according to individual requirements, up to a maximum of 100-300 mg per day. Occasionally, under supervision, the drug can be taken twice a day rather than four times a day.

adverse effects

If Apresoline is taken along with a sympathetic blocking drug such as Aldomet or Inderal, it has relatively few side effects apart from a sensation of lightheadedness on moving suddenly. In the absence of a sympathetic blocking drug, Apresoline can, because of its dilating effect on the blood vessels, cause an increase in heart rate. This can be a problem in the presence of other heart conditions, such as angina pectoris, because of the extra work required of the heart. Other side effects may include occasional headache, nausea and flushing. At high doses, some patients develop lupus erythematosus, an arthritis-like disorder characterized by a facial rash and joint and muscle pain, which usually necessitates the discontinuation of the drug. Other allergic reactions may also occur.

precautions

Apresoline should not be used in pregnant or nursing women and should be used with caution in persons with angina pectoris or previous stroke.

drug interactions

Other drugs for high blood pressure, diuretics like Aldactone, Lasix and hydrochlorothiazide, and MAO inhibitor drugs like Marplan, Nardil and Parnate can all increase Apresoline's effect on blood pressure.

see essays

Drugs for High Blood Pressure. Diuretics.

Aristocort Cream and Ointment

generic name

> triamcinolone (available by generic name)

action and uses

A commonly used topical preparation of a synthetic

127

corticosteroid, or cortisone-like drug. It is used primarily because of its antiinflammatory effects in the treatment of many types of skin disorders such as psoriasis, certain types of neurodermatitis and a variety of other conditions which are not infected. In many cases, the effects are dramatic. Because it also retards formation of scar tissue, it can prevent scarring.

adult dosage

The 0.025 – 0.5% preparation is applied sparingly 3 – 4 times daily. It is available in ointment, and cream in several strengths, depending upon where it is used.

adverse effects

If the preparation is not used for long periods or on infected areas, there are virtually no important adverse effects; however, if the preparations are used for long intervals on the face, they can cause eruptions and redness. If Aristocort preparations are used for long periods on a large portion of the body, the corticosteroid can be absorbed and get into the body. This can cause weight gain, ulcers or stomach upset, decreased resistance to infection and stress, and can be quite hazardous. If used on an infected area of the skin it can help the infection spread, and it can be very hazardous if used for any viral skin lesions such as herpes (cold sores), shingles or chickenpox.

precautions

Do not use without a physician's specific instructions, and use only on affected areas. Do not use on a skin area which appears infected without consulting a physician.

drug interactions

No significant interactions will occur although other topical preparations placed on the same skin area may interfere with effects.

see essays

Steroids or Cortisone-like Drugs. Drugs for Skin and Local Disorders.

Artane

generic name

trihexyphenidyl

action and uses

A drug used to treat tremor and rigidity of muscles, particularly associated with Parkinson's disease. Parkinson's disease is thought to be caused by an imbalance of nervous activity in the brain. Artane helps correct this imbalance presumably by blocking the activity of cholinergic nerves; thus, the drug is an anticholinergic. It may also relax muscles directly. It is only moderately effective in some people, so a new drug, levodopa, is now far more widely used to treat Parkinsonism than drugs such as Artane. If the two different drugs are used together in lower doses, fewer side effects are often experienced. Artane, and a similar drug, Cogentin, are also used in drug-caused Parkinson's disease, as seen when the major tranquilizers are used.

adult dosage The dosage varies according to the response of the patient. Initially, the dose is 1 mg daily. This is increased every 3 to 5 days by 2 mg to a total of 10 mg, or sometimes even 15 mg daily. With high doses, it is best to take Artane in three or four divided doses with meals. When optimum dosage has been established, it may be substituted by the long-acting Sequels, which are taken usually as a single dose after breakfast.

adverse effects These are common to all anticholinergic drugs (such as atropine) and include dry mouth, constipation and retention of urine. Blurring of vision, nausea, dizziness or nervousness may also occur.

precautions Artane may increase visual problems in persons with glaucoma, bladder difficulties in those with prostate trouble, and make expectoration difficult in those with chronic lung disease.

drug interactions Artane adds to the effects of other anticholinergic drugs such as antihistamines, antispasmodics, cough/cold medicines and tricyclic antidepressants. This can cause dry mouth, difficulty urinating, constipation and blurred vision.

see essay *Drugs for Parkinson's Disease.*

Aspirin (acetylsalicylic acid)

trade names

ASA, Ecotrin, Measurin

action and uses Aspirin is still one of the most effective drugs for the relief of mild to moderate pain. It is also useful in bringing down fever, and because it reduces inflammation, has proved itself a most effective drug in the treatment of arthritis. Recently, aspirin has also been cited for its anticoagulant effects: it helps prevent blood clotting by reducing the stickiness of certain blood cells called platelets. Its primary use, however, is as a pain reliever and anti-inflammatory agent.

Originally, the word "Aspirin" (based on the German word for salicylic acid, *Spirsaure*) was used only by the Bayer Drug Company as a brand name for their product.

129

Since then, the drug has become so popular and widely used that "aspirin" has become virtually synonymous with the acetylsalicylic acid is stands for.

Today, aspirin is not only marketed on its own, but also in over a hundred different combination drugs for everything from headaches and hangovers to strained and aching muscles and heavy colds. Alka-Seltzer, APC, Anacin, Ascriptin, Bufferin, Cope, Coricidin, Darvon Compound, Dristin, Empirin Compound, Equagesic, Excedrin, Fiorinal, Norgesic, Percodan, Phenaphen and Vanquish are just a few of the aspirin-containing compounds in popular use. It is important to be aware of the aspirin content in all these and many other cold and headache remedies available over the counter, because however commonplace and "harmless" aspirin may seem, it *is* a drug and can produce side effects, allergic reactions and harmful interactions with other drugs.

It is also interesting to note that, despite all the claims made by the various "name brands", plain ordinary aspirin has often proved itself as good or better for the relief of any type of pain as any other non-narcotic pain reliever on the market. Many of the combination drugs are a good deal more expensive, with the extra money going for various additions or refinements of dubious value. In the case of Ascriptin, Bufferin and similar drugs you may be paying for the addition of "buffers" or antacids to prevent stomach irritation, though the antacids are present in quantities too small to be very helpful in preventing irritation. Some aspirin-containing pain relievers are "coated" to keep them from irritating the stomach: unfortunately, this also means that they usually take considerably longer to work, or are never absorbed into the body! Alka-Seltzer gets around the problem of gastric irritation by including sodium bicarbonate (a well-known antacid) with aspirin. The presence of sodium bicarbonate, however, limits Alka-Seltzer's all-round usefulness, (for example, the sodium can cause fluid retention) and, of course, also raises the price of the preparation.

adult dosage

Customarily available in 300 mg or 5-grain tablets, aspirin is usually taken with lots of water in doses of 600 mg or 10 grains (two tablets' worth) every 3 to 6 hours as needed for pain. For treatment of arthritis, it is taken in somewhat higher doses (frequently 2 to 4 tablets every 4 hours) on a regular basis under a doctor's supervision. Aspirin may deteriorate if damp, and should be discarded if it develops a strong acid or vinegar odor.

adverse effects
Aspirin may irritate the stomach lining, causing nausea, vomiting, pain and even bleeding, especially when taken in higher doses, or frequently. Even when taken on an occasional basis, aspirin should always be taken with plenty of fluid to help prevent stomach irritation. Too much aspirin can also produce dizziness, mental confusion, and a ringing in the ears. Some people are allergic to aspirin, and may develop skin rashes or symptoms like those of asthma or hay fever.

precautions
Aspirin and drugs containing it should be avoided by those with peptic ulcer and anyone taking anticoagulants except under specific instructions. Those who have allergic sinusitis or asthma may have an allergy to aspirin. Because this common drug is a major cause of accidental overdose in children, it should always be kept out of their reach.

drug interactions
Aspirin adds to the effects of anticoagulant drugs such as Coumadin and Dicumarol to increase the risk of bleeding. Taken in conjunction with cortisone-like drugs, it increases the chances of developing ulcers. It may interact with Diabinese and other diabetes drugs to cause a dangerous fall in blood sugar.

see essay
Drugs for Pain with Inflammation.

Atarax

generic name

> hydroxyzine

action and uses
An antihistamine which is primarily promoted for its anti-anxiety and sedating actions. It has a chemical structure similar to other antihistamines such as Marezine, which are used for motion sickness, and it is essentially identical to the drug Vistaril. It is also used on occasion as an antihistamine and in the treatment of conditions which cause itching of the skin.

adult dosage
Because sensitivity to its effect varies, the dose ranges from 25 to 100 mg 2 to 3 times a day.

adverse effects
Excessive sedation or decreased mental alertness may create a significant problem. Other side effects are relatively unusual.

precautions
Atarax may interfere with driving or operating machinery. It should not be used by pregnant, potentially pregnant or nursing women.

drug interactions
Atarax is additive to other drugs causing sedation such

as sleeping pills, tranquilizers, alcohol and narcotics such as morphine; these combinations should be avoided unless greater sedation is required.

see essays

Antihistamines. Minor Tranquilizers.

Atromid-S

generic name

clofibrate

action and uses

A drug used to lower high levels of cholesterol (fat) in the blood. It is believed to help prevent coronary heart disease and other circulatory disease by reducing the accumulation of fatty deposits that line the walls of the arteries and endanger the normal flow of blood to the heart and elsewhere. However, it is probable that exercise and weight reduction, a balanced low fat diet and giving up smoking may be even more effective than this or other currently available drugs in the battle against the build-up of fat in the arteries.

adult dosage

Usually 1 – 2 grams per day in divided doses.

adverse effects

Atromid-S may cause a wide variety of adverse effects, the most common being gastrointestinal upset, including reactivation of ulcers. Less frequently, it can cause reversible liver damage, blood cell abnormalities, irregular heart rhythms, various skin rashes, and flu-like symptoms.

precautions

Atromid-S should not be taken by patients with impaired liver or kidney function. It should not be used by pregnant or potentially pregnant women.

drug interactions

Atromid-S may markedly increase the effects of the anticoagulant drug, Coumadin, thus increasing the risk of bleeding. It can also increase the effects of oral antidiabetic and possibly other drugs.

see essay

Drugs used to Prevent or Treat Circulation Problems.

Azo Gantrisin

generic ingredients

antibacterial = sulfisoxazole painkiller = phenazopyridine hydrochloride

action and uses

A fixed combination drug used to treat infections of the kidney, bladder and urinary tract, including cystitis. Azo Gantrisin combines a sulfonamide or "sulfa" drug with a pain killer. Phenazopyridine is a pain killer which acts specifically on the urinary tract. Azo Gantrisin is therefore particularly suitable for treating painful urinary infections.

adult dosage
Usually 4 to 6 tablets initially, followed by 2 tablets 4 times per day for 3 days. Treatment is usually continued with Gantrisin tablets.

adverse effects
This drug may sometimes cause nausea, vomiting or other gastrointestinal symptoms as well as headaches or dizziness. Like all sulfa drugs, Azo Gantrisin may cause allergic reactions such as rashes, as well as very serious, life-threatening reactions with fever, severe rash, and kidney failure. The most common but harmless side effect is the change of color of the urine to an orange-red, due to the "azo" dye. This is harmless (though it can stain underwear) and disappears when the drug is stopped. Rashes or other allergies may also occur due to this dye.

precautions
It is always important to drink plenty of water while taking this drug to prevent crystal formation in the kidney. If any fever, nausea or rash occur after starting the drug, it should be discontinued and the doctor notified. It should be avoided in persons with severe kidney disease or G6PD deficiency (a congenital red blood cell disease). As in the treatment of all infections, it is important to take the drug for the full time recommended to prevent recurrence of the infection. Pregnant, potentially pregnant and nursing women should avoid the drug if possible.

drug interactions
As with many sulfa drugs, Azo Gantrisin may increase the effect of oral antidiabetic drugs (to cause low blood sugar) and Dilantin, Butazolidin, and phenobarbital to increase the likelihood of toxicity to these drugs.

see essay
Drugs to Treat Infections.

Benadryl
Benadryl Elixir

generic name

diphenhydramine (available by generic name)

action and uses
A popular drug used to treat allergies, rashes, and itching of the skin. Benadryl is also sometimes used as a sedative. It is an antihistamine which blocks the effects of a substance (histamine) released in the body during allergic reactions. When histamine is released it causes itching, swelling and redness. Benadryl is useful in hay fever, hives, redness of the eyes or allergic conjunctivitis. It is not generally used in allergic asthma. It is sometimes used as a sleeping pill, particularly in older persons, and when

effective it is relatively useful and safe.

adult dosage

Usually 25-50 mg every six to twelve hours for allergic problems. The dose varies according to the sedative effects. For night time use the usual dosage is 50 mg. It comes in tablet, capsule and elixir form.

adverse effects

The most common side effect of Benadryl is drowsiness which occurs in some people but not in others. Other side effects are not common.

precautions

When drowsiness occurs it is advisable to avoid driving or operating fast moving machinery. It should be avoided by pregnant or potentially pregnant women and nursing mothers.

drug interactions

Benadryl is additive to any other sedative or tranquilizer, or alcohol, especially in those people who are susceptible to its sedative effects. It also interacts with drugs such as Pro-Banthine and Librax to increase the likelihood of side effects such as blurred vision, dry mouth and difficulty urinating.

see essays

Antihistamines. Sleeping Pills.

Bendectin

generic
ingredients

antihistamine/antinauseant = doxylamine
vitamin = pyridoxine (vitamin B_6)

action and uses

A combination of an antihistamine and vitamin B_6 promoted for a nausea often experienced in early pregnancy. Bendectin has not been shown to produce any harmful effects on the baby if taken during pregnancy, although this remains controversial. Like many antihistamine drugs, Bendectin has a prominent antinauseant effect, but it also has other antihistamine effects as well. The vitamin B_6 is present to help correct any existing vitamin deficiency, but it is doubtful whether this is of any practical value.

adult dosage

Bendectin is supplied as tablets containing 10 mg of each constituent in a special coating designed to delay release of the antihistamine. The dose is 2 tablets taken at bedtime.

adverse effects

Bendectin has the same side effects as other antihistamine drugs – namely sedation, and occasionally dry mouth, blurring of vision, and possibly difficulty with passing urine, or wheezing. Some people feel restless instead of drowsy, and find it difficult to sleep.

precautions

Because of the possible sedative effect, driving or operating hazardous machinery should be avoided when taking Bendectin. In those who suffer from asthma or glaucoma, Bendectin may not be indicated.

drug interactions The effects of Bendectin are additive with sedative drugs, sleeping tablets and alcohol, and to the antispasmodic effect of drugs such as Pro-Banthine and Librax.

see essays *Drugs for Nausea, Stomach Upset and Ulcers. Antihistamines. Vitamins and Minerals.*

Bentyl

generic name

> antispasmodic = dicyclomine hydrochloride
> (available by generic name)

Bentyl with Phenobarbital

generic ingredients

> antispasmodic = dicyclomine hydrochloride
> minor tranquilizer = phenobarbital

action and uses Drugs used to relieve spasm or tightness of the muscles of the stomach and intestines. Bentyl is an antispasmodic-anticholinergic drug which acts to produce a relaxing effect directly on the stomach. It is used in the treatment of stomach and duodenal ulcers and other gastrointestinal spasm. The preparation with phenobarbital is like many similar products combining an antispasmodic with a minor tranquilizer on the assumption that the relief of anxiety will relieve the symptoms as well. Single antispasmodic drugs are likely to be as effective.

adult dosage Usually 10-20 mg three or four times a day. When combined with phenobarbital each tablet or capsule and each teaspoonful of syrup also contains 15 mg of phenobarbital.

adverse effects The antispasmodic component may cause a dry mouth, difficulty in urinating (particularly in the elderly), blurred vision and constipation. It can also cause drying of bronchial secretions. In Bentyl with Phenobarbital, phenobarbital may cause allergic reactions such as skin rash and, infrequently, sedation.

precautions Bentyl should be used with caution by people who have glaucoma, prostate trouble, hiatus hernia or chronic lung disease. The phenobarbital may cause drowsiness and driving or operating machinery may be hazardous.

drug dependence Phenobarbital may cause dependence if used over long periods.

drug interactions The antispasmodics can have additive effects when taken with antihistamines, cough/cold medicines and tricyclic antidepressants to cause excessive dry mouth, constipation and occasional bladder problems. The phenobarbital can decrease the effect of the anticoagulant, Coumadin, and might potentially add to the effects of other sedatives, tranquilizers or alcohol.

see essay

Drugs for Nausea, Stomach Upset and Ulcers.

Benylin Cough Syrup

generic ingredients

antihistamine = diphenhydramine expectorants = ammonium chloride, sodium citrate miscellaneous = chloroform, menthol, alcohol

action and uses

A widely prescribed cough mixture containing an antihistamine which is also believed to have a mild cough suppressant effect, and expectorants, which are believed to help liquefy bronchial secretions. In fact, the effectiveness of this and other similar cough syrups is difficult to establish.

adult dosage

Usually two teaspoonfuls every 4 hours, not to exceed 12 teaspoons per 24 hours.

adverse effects

The antihistamines can cause drowsiness, and less frequently, dizziness. The expectorants can sometimes cause nausea.

precautions

If drowsiness occurs, it may interfere with driving and operating machinery. Benylin should be avoided by pregnant or potentially pregnant women or nursing mothers.

drug interactions

The antihistamines in Benylin can add to the effects of alcohol, tranquilizers and sleeping pills, as well as antispasmodic anticholinergic drugs such as Pro-Banthine or Librax. Because of the alcohol, Benylin can cause a hazardous interaction if Flagyl or Antabuse is also taken.

see essays

Drugs for Coughs and Colds. Antihistamines.

Brompheniramine (generic name). See DIMETANE.

Butabarbital (generic name). See BUTISOL.

Butazolidin

generic

phenylbutazone

Butazolidin Alka

generic ingredients

anti-inflammatory drug = phenylbutazone antacids =aluminum hydroxide, magnesium trisilicate

action and uses
A drug used to reduce inflammation, especially in the joints. Butazolidin relieves the painful symptoms of inflammation but does not cure the disease which causes the inflammation. It is not known how it works. It is not a steroid hormone and is not related to steroids, although its anti-inflammatory actions are similar. Because it has very serious side effects, it is used only when milder drugs, such as aspirin, do not relieve the symptoms of inflammation. It is useful in treating isolated severe joint pains of inflamed tendons and joints, occasionally for acute gout, and for the acute flare-ups of rheumatoid arthritis.

adult dosage
The dosage of Butazolidin varies from person to person and must be determined by the physician for each individual case. It is available in 100 mg tablets, and the daily dose ranges from 300-600 mg, usually taken in divided doses with meals or milk.

adverse effects
While Butazolidin is an effective and useful drug it is also a dangerous and poisonous drug. Many severe reactions occur, particularly it it is used for longer than 7 days, especially in persons over the age of 60. It may poison the bone marrow and prevent the body from producing both red and white blood cells, thereby causing anemia and loss of resistance to infection. If such a reaction occurs the effects may be irreversible if the drug is not stopped immediately. Hives, skin rashes, itching and sores in and around the mouth can be signs of serious reactions to the drug and should be reported to the physician immediately. Butazolidin also may cause stomach upsets, nausea, vomiting and indigestion, though this may be avoided by taking it with meals. It can also cause liver damage and fluid retention.

precautions
Butazolidin should not be used by children under age 14, pregnant, potentially pregnant or nursing women. It should never be used for more than 7 days in any person over the age of 60 unless specifically ordered by, and discussed with, a physician and should be followed with regular blood counts. It should be used cautiously in persons who have stomach or intestinal trouble or ulcers.

drug interactions
Butazolidin interacts with many drugs, including

antidiabetic drugs, other antiinflammatory drugs such as Motrin, sulfa drugs, Dilantin and Coumadin, increasing the risk of toxicity of each.

see essay

Drugs for Pain with Inflammation.

Butisol

generic name

butabarbital (available by generic name)

action and uses

A barbiturate similar to Seconal and Nembutal. Butisol is chiefly used as a sleeping pill, although it is occasionally used as a daytime sedative to relieve anxiety and tension. It takes effect 15-30 minutes after being taken and this effect lasts 5-6 hours. When used as a sleeping medication Butisol decreases the time it takes to go to sleep but it suppresses dreaming. After a few days, tolerance can develop and it is necessary to increase the dosage to produce the same sleep inducing effect. Some of the effects of Butisol may last longer than 5-6 hours, such as a hangover which may occur the morning after taking the drug.

adult dosage

For sleep the usual dose is 50-100 mg at bedtime. If used in the daytime for relief of anxiety and tension the usual dose is 30 mg, 2 to 4 times per day.

adverse effects

When used as a sleeping pill Butisol may cause a hangover effect the following morning. It may also cause a feeling of depression and tiredness, together with nausea, vomiting and diarrhea. If Butisol is withdrawn after several weeks of use withdrawal symptoms may appear. There is often a tendency for increased dreaming and even nightmares. There may be insomnia (difficulty in sleeping) and nervousness. If the dose has been high (over 400 mg per day) seizures may occur. All these effects are due to the withdrawal of the drug. Other mild side effects of the drug include allergic skin reactions, upset stomach and muscular aches. Butisol can suppress breathing in persons with severe lung diseases.

precautions

Butisol and other barbiturates have long been a major cause of suicidal and accidental drug overdose and death. If taken in high doses they can be lethal. Barbiturates can be particularly dangerous if taken with alcohol, or other tranquilizers.

drug
dependence

If used for longer than 7 to 10 days, "tolerance" to Butisol may develop. If this occurs dependence on the drug may develop and if it is suddenly discontinued withdrawal symptoms may occur. Therefore, it must be stopped slowly if it has been used for a long time. Because of this problem, as well as its known abuse, the prescribing of Butisol is restricted.

drug interactions   Butisol can interact with many other drugs, particularly the anticoagulant Coumadin to decrease its effect.

Barbiturates add to the effects of other tranquilizers, sleeping pills and alcohol. The combination with any of these drugs can be very hazardous, causing suppression of breathing and even death.

see essays   *Minor Tranquilizers. Sleeping Pills.*

Catapres

generic name

clonidine

action and uses   A drug used to treat moderately or severely high blood pressure, usually only if other drugs such as Aldomet or Inderal are ineffective. It acts in the brain to block the sympathetic nervous system and cause relaxation or dilation of the arteries. Most commonly it is used with a diuretic ("water pill").

adult dosage   Initially, 0.1 to 0.2 mg twice daily, with gradual dosage adjustments until the desired blood pressure response is obtained. The maintenance dosage from then on is usually 0.2 to 0.8 mg daily in 2-3 divided doses. The drug's effect on blood pressure will be felt 30-60 minutes after it has been taken, and lasts 6-8 hours. The last dose of the day is usually taken just before retiring, to insure adequate overnight blood pressure control.

adverse effects   Catapres may cause dry mouth, constipation, sleepiness, dizziness, headache and fatigue. These side effects tend to disappear as therapy with the drug continues. The major problem with Catapres is that sudden discontinuation of the drug can cause an equally sudden often severe rise in blood pressure, which may be accompanied by headache, nervousness and agitation as well as by more severe symptoms. Discontinuation of Catapres should therefore be done slowly and cautiously under a doctor's supervision.

precautions   The sedation caused by Catapres may interfere with driving or operating machinery. Catapres should be used with caution by pregnant or potentially pregnant women.

drug interactions Over sedation can result from combining Catapres with alcohol, sedatives, sleeping pills, tranquilizers, antihistamines or pain relievers, whether narcotic or non-narcotic.

see essays *Drugs for High Blood Pressure. Diuretics.*

Chloral Hydrate

trade names

Noctec, Somnos, Kessodrate

action and uses A common sleeping pill. It is often used in elderly people since it is believed to be better tolerated and less likely to cause excitement. In lower doses, it does not suppress dreaming (REM sleep) like most sleeping pills. The value of this is unknown, but lack of REM sleep has been shown to cause irritability and anxiety. The effectiveness of the drug in producing sleep decreases over time as tolerance develops.

adult dosage 0.5 to 1.0 gram at bedtime, taken with water or milk to decrease stomach irritation.

adverse effects Like other sleeping pills, chloral hydrate can cause a morning hangover. It can also cause dizziness, depression and very occasionally excitement. It can cause stomach irritation. Allergic reactions can rarely occur.

precautions This drug should not be used by pregnant or potentially pregnant women or nursing mothers. The sedating effect may interfere with driving or operating machinery.

drug dependence Chloral hydrate can cause psychological and physical dependence and withdrawal symptoms can occur if discontinued after prolonged use.

drug interactions Chloral hydrate can add dangerously to the sedative effects of alcohol, and minor tranquilizers. It can also alter the effects of the anticoagulant Coumadin.

see essay *Sleeping Pills.*

Chlordiazepoxide (generic name). See LIBRIUM.

Chlorothiazide (generic name). See DIURIL.

Chlorpheniramine (generic name).
See CHLOR-TRIMETON, POLARAMINE, TELDRIN.

Chlorpromazine (generic name). See THORAZINE.

Chlor-Trimeton

generic name

chlorpheniramine (available by generic name)

action and uses

A commonly prescribed antihistamine which is frequently used to treat allergic conditions, especially allergic rhinitis, sinusitis or conjunctivitis (redness of the eye). It shares the effects of most other antihistamines by blocking the effects of histamine and thus can decrease itching of the skin due to allergies, hives or rashes. It also can sometimes have a sedating effect, although it is not customarily used for this. It is not useful for treatment for asthma. It is usually much less expensive in generic form, as chlorpheniramine.

adult dosage

Chlor-Trimeton is available in oral tablets and liquid forms and for injections. The usual oral dose is 4 mg, 2 to 6 times daily, or one 8 mg Repetab twice daily as needed for treatment of allergic conditions.

adverse effects

Although possibly less frequently than with some other antihistamines, Chlor-Trimeton may also cause significant sedation is some people. Other side effects are relatively rare, but can include dry mouth, blurred vision, or difficulty in urinating, especially in older persons or those with glaucoma or prostate trouble.

drug interactions

Chlor-Trimeton is additive to other sedative or tranquilizing drugs and alcohol. It is also additive to other antispasmodic drugs used to treat ulcers or stomach problems, such as Pro-Banthine or Librax, to cause excessive dry mouth, constipation and difficulty in urinating.

precautions

The sedative effects may interfere with driving or operating machinery. This drug should be used with caution in those with glaucoma or prostate trouble. It should be avoided by pregnant or potentially pregnant women and nursing mothers.

see essay

Antihistamines.

Cleocin

generic name

clindamycin

action and uses

An antibiotic used to treat infections caused by specific bacteria. Cleocin is particularly effective in treating infections caused by the bacterium *Bacteroides*, which most commonly causes serious pelvic and abdominal infections.

141

It can cause serious adverse reactions and should only be used for infections for which other drugs are not effective. It is not used to treat infections such as colds and bronchitis.

adult dosage Usually 150–300 mg every six hours.

adverse effects The most common side effect of Cleocin is diarrhea. This may be mild, but in some cases may be severe and may result in a serious inflammation of the large intestine which can even result in death. Some people may develop skin rashes when taking the drug.

precautions Pregnant, potentially pregnant and nursing women should use caution in taking this drug. Use of Cleocin requires careful medical supervision. If diarrhea occurs, the physician should be notified.

drug interactions Clindamycin and erythromycin may be antagonistic to one another and thus should not be used together.

see essay *Drugs to Treat Infections.*

Codeine

action and uses A very common oral narcotic for treatment of moderate to severe pain. It is frequently combined with other pain relievers such as aspirin, acetaminophen and/or phenacetin in preparations such as Empirin with codeine, or Tylenol with codeine. Its use alone requires special restricted prescriptions.

adult dosage This varies with severity of pain and need. It is usually 15-30 mg every 4 to 6 hours for severe pain.

adverse effects A certain number of people suffer nausea when taking codeine, although this is not a true allergy. Constipation almost always occurs if use continues for more than one or two days. Some experience dizziness or unusual dreams.

precautions Codeine should be used only when less potent pain relievers are not effective. It must be used with caution in persons with chronic lung disease.

drug dependence Codeine can cause physiological dependence and if discontinued after prolonged use, withdrawal symptoms can occur.

drug interactions Codeine can add to the sedative and breathing depression effects of sedatives, tranquilizers and alcohol. It can also add to the constipating effect of many antispasmodic drugs and antihistamines.

see essay *Narcotic Pain Relievers.*

Combid

generic ingredients	antispasmodic = isopropamide major tranquilizer = prochlorperazine

action and uses A fixed combination drug used in the treatment of stomach and intestinal disorders. Combid is widely used to treat ulcers, irritable and spastic colon, and colitis. Like many similar drugs it combines an antispasmodic-anticholinergic drug, which reduces secretions from the stomach and decreases tightness (spasm) of the stomach muscles, with a major tranquilizer to relieve anxiety and tension. The major tranquilizer also has the effect of reducing nausea and vomiting and stopping hiccoughs. Apparently, it is assumed that many bowel conditions are associated with anxiety and can be relieved by a tranquilizer. Whether this combination is really more effective than an antispasmodic alone is not known.

adult dosage Usually one capsule every 10 to 12 hours.

adverse effects Effects due to both ingredients can occur. The antispasmodic can cause dry mouth, blurred vision and difficulty in urinating, especially in older people. The major tranquilizer can infrequently cause drowsiness, various allergic reactions, liver or blood cell abnormalities, but also can cause neurological reactions, such as parkinsonian reactions (tremor, rigid extremities) and acute spasm of the neck and jaw muscles (the latter is more common in young people).

precautions Combid should not be taken by pregnant or potentially pregnant or nursing women, particularly since the major tranquilizer can be very hazardous for infants and children.

This combination should be used with caution in those with glaucoma, prostate trouble, and chronic lung disease. Those with a history of sensitivity to phenothiazines should not take this drug. If drowsiness occurs, driving or operating machinery may be hazardous.

drug interactions The antispasmodic can add to the effects (and cause dry mouth, bladder difficulties and constipation) of antihistamines, cough/cold medicines and tricyclic antidepressants. The major tranquilizer can enhance the effects of alcohol, and other sedating drugs, and block the effect of Ismelin, a drug for high blood pressure.

see essays *Drugs for Nausea, Stomach Upset, and Ulcers. Major Tranquilizers.*

Compazine

generic name

> prochlorperazine

action and uses

A member of the major tranquilizer group of drugs which is primarily used to treat nausea and vomiting. Ideally, it should only be used for this if the cause is known and the symptoms are not controlled by less hazardous drugs. The same antinausea action is also used to stop hiccoughs. It is commonly used to stop nausea after surgery. It is also commonly used combined with an antispasmodic drug in Combid Spansules. Although it shares the antipsychotic effects of all phenothiazines such as Thorazine, it is only infrequently used to treat thought disorders such as schizophrenia.

adult dosage

5-10 mg orally or by injection every 6-8 hours for nausea. The Spansule and suppository forms are given every 12 hours as needed. Dosage should be individualized. Lower doses are usually required in older patients.

adverse effects

Compazine may cause a dry mouth, constipation, and in younger adults there is more likelihood of acute reaction expressed by grimacing and spasms of the neck and facial muscles (relieved by drugs such as Cogentin or Benadryl). Some persons may experience hypersensitivity reactions such as jaundice, rashes, or a fall in the white blood count. Prolonged use can result in a Parkinson's syndrome of trembling of the hands, rigidity of the arms and legs, and loss of facial expression.

precautions

Compazine should not be taken by pregnant women or potentially pregnant or nursing women, particularly since this drug can be very hazardous for infants and children. Persons who have had allergic reactions to Thorazine or phenothiazines should not take this drug.

drug interactions

Oversedation may occur if Compazine is used with alcohol, tranquilizers or sleeping pills, and antihistamines. It can counteract the effect of some antihypertensive drugs such as Ismelin.

see essays

Drugs for Nausea, Stomach Upset and Ulcer. Major Tranquilizers.

Cordran cream, ointment and lotion

generic name

> flurandrenolide (available by generic name)

action and uses | A commonly used topical preparation of a synthetic corticosteriod, or cortisone-like drug. It is used primarily because of its anti-inflammatory effects in the treatment of many types of skin disorders such as psoriasis, certain types of neurodermatitis and a variety of other conditions which are not infected. In many cases, the effects are dramatic. Because it retards formation of scar tissue, it can also prevent scarring.

adult dosage | The 0.025 – 0.05% preparation is applied sparingly 2-3 times daily. It is available in ointments, lotions, and creams in several strengths, depending upon where it is to be used.

adverse effects | If the preparation is not used for long periods or on infected areas, there are virtually no important adverse effects; however, if the preparations are used for long intervals on the face, they can cause eruptions and redness. If Cordran preparations are used for long periods on a large portion of the body, the corticosteroid can be absorbed and get into the body. This can cause weight gain, ulcers or stomach upset, decreased resistance to infection and stress, and can be quite hazardous. If used on an infected area of the skin it can help the infection spread, and it can be very hazardous if used for any viral skin lesions such as herpes (cold sores), shingles or chickenpox.

precautions | Do not use without a physician's specific instructions, and use only on affected areas. Do not use on a skin area which appears infected without consulting a physician.

drug interactions | No significant interactions will occur although other topical preparations placed on the same skin area may interfere with effects.

see essays | *Steroids or Cortisone-like Drugs. Drugs for Skin and Local Disorders.*

Cortisporin

generic ingredients |

```
antibiotics = polymixin B
              neomycin
              gramicidin
   steroid = hydrocortisone
```

action and uses | A combination product used to treat local infections of the skin, eyes and ears. Cortisporin combines three antibiotics and a steroid or cortisone-like drug. Each of the antibiotics acts against different types of bacteria. The steroid acts to

145

reduce inflammation and irritation. The ointment is used in a variety of skin irritations with mild infection; the eye and ear drops for similar local problems in these areas. This type of mixture has been criticized because it represents "shotgun" therapy when one specific ingredient may often be adequate.

adult dosage
Available as a cream, ointment, lotion and suspension, as well as ear and eye drops which are usually applied 2 to 4 times per day.

adverse effects
Allergy to any of the ingredients of Cortisporin may occur and skin conditions may worsen rather than improve. This is particularly true of neomycin which has a high rate of allergic reactions. The steroid may rarely worsen infections, especially if caused by a virus, as in shingles. Serious adverse effects can occur from all the ingredients if the preparation is used on large areas for a long time, due to absorption. Also, resistant bacteria or fungi can appear and cause reinfection.

precautions
Cortisporin should not be used over large parts of the body at any one time. It should not be used to treat the sores of "cold sore," or on smallpox vaccinations or chickenpox sores.

drug interactions
If properly used, drug interactions are not a problem.

see essays
Drugs to Treat Infections. Drugs for Skin and Local Disorders. Steroids or Cortisone-like Drugs.

Coumadin

generic name

warfarin

action and uses
An anticoagulant drug used to treat patients who have already developed, or are in danger of developing, a life-threatening clot (thrombosis) in an artery, a vein, or the heart itself. Although often referred to as a "blood thinner," Coumadin actually works by slowing down the time it takes the blood to clot. Coumadin is a very effective drug, but it operates within an extremely narrow safety margin: if the dosage is too low, there is the danger of a blood clot forming; if the dosage is too high, there is the opposite danger of a hemorrhage.

adult dosage
Coumadin is usually taken just once a day. The exact dosage necessars to prevent clotting while keeping the possibility of excessive bleeding to a minimun is highly individualized and is determined by regular laboratory tests

of the prothrombin time. Coumadin tablets come in six color-coded strengths: the 2 mg tablet is lavender; the 2.5 mg tablet ie orange; the 5 mg tablet is peach; the 7.5 mg tablet is yellow; the 10 mg tablet is white; and the 25 mg tablet is red.

adverse effects

Excessive bleeding is the most serious and common side effect of Coumadin. Because the drug works to slow down the clotting mechanism, even a small cut or internal injury can lead to uncontrolled bleeding. Patients on Coumadin should inform their doctor right away if they notice any of the following warning signals: red or dark brown urine; red or blackbowel movements; increased or prolonged menstrual bleeding; continued bleeding from minor cuts, nose or gums; prolonged stomachache, headache, or backache; or the sudden appearance of black and blue marks. Skin rash, nausea or diarrhea are among the other, far less frequent side effects possible with the drug.

precautions

The narrow margin of safety of Coumadin can be adversely affected by a number of other drugs; it is *vital* for the patient on Coumadin to know what they are. (See below). Patients on an anticoagulant like Coumadin must be under close medical supervision: they should also carry a card and or wear some identification indicating that they are on this drug in case of accident. Naturally, they should inform their dentist or any other health professional they see for treatment that they are taking Coumadin, and report to their own doctor right away if pregnancy is discovered or suspected, or if any illness, infection or injury occurs.

drug interactions

Potentially serious interactions are possible when Coumadin is taken concurrently with *any* of the following: aspirin and all medications containing it (including the scores of different preparations for headache, hangover, aching muscles, and cold symptoms), many of the drugs for arthritis, tranquilizers, sleeping pills and sedatives, birth control pills, cortisone-like drugs, thyroid gland supplements, drugs for diabetes, drugs to lower cholesterol, antibiotics, antidepressants, antihistamines, digitalis drugs, drugs for epilepsy, alcohol, leafy green vegetables, and the vitamin K in multivitamin tablets. All these, as well as numerous other drugs, can affect Coumadin's action in the body. Some increase its anticoagulant effect, others decrease it, but so dangerous are the results of either interaction that it is unwise to take any other medication, whether prescribed by a medical professional or just purchased over the counter, without first consulting the doctor.

see essay

Anticoagulants.

Cyclandelate (generic name). See CYCLOSPASMOL.

Cyclospasmol

generic name

cyclandelate (available by generic name)

action and uses

A drug promoted and used to improve the circulation in the arms, legs or brain. Known as a "vasodilator", it acts in normal persons to relax the blood vessels, causing the vessels to expand and let more blood through. Its effects are generally unproven or minimal in abnormal circulatory states but it is still used in conditions caused by the spastic decrease in the size of the blood vessels, including nocturnal leg cramps, intermittent cramping of leg and foot muscles on exercise, and Raynaud's phenomenon.

adult dosage

The initial dose is usually 1200-1600 mg per day in 4 divided doses, taken with meals and an antacid, and at bedtime. If a favorable effect is noted, the dosage may be reduced to 400-800 mg per day.

adverse effects

Cyclospasmol may cause stomach upset, headache, dizziness or heart palpitation, flushing of the face, and a feeling of weakness.

precautions

Cyclandelate should be used with caution by patients with coronary heart disease, or ulcer disease. It should be avoided if possible by pregnant or potentially pregnant women.

see essay

Drugs to Prevent or Treat Circulation Problems.

Dalmane

generic name

flurazepam

action and uses

A minor tranquilizer which is very popular as a nightime sedative (sleeping medication). Dalmane is closely related to a group of tranquilizers which includes Librium and Valium and their actions are very similar. Dalmane decreases the time it takes to fall asleep, decreases the number of awakenings, and increases the total length of sleep without stopping dreaming. Barbiturates and most other sleeping pills tend to suppress dreaming and Dalmane is considered better in this respect, although Dalmane blocks other parts of the sleep cycle, so that the sleep produced is still different from normal.

adult dosage Usually 15 to 30 mg at bedtime.

adverse effects In some people Dalmane causes a "hangover" in the morning. It can also cause depression and dizziness. When Dalmane is stopped after regular use for three weeks or more, there is usually an increase in the deep stage of sleep and often nightmares are experienced. These probably represent withdrawal symptoms.

precautions There is a possibility that minor tranquilizers may cause birth defects and the manufacturers therefore warn against the use of Dalmane in pregnant and potentially pregnant women. In some cases, the sedation may interfere with working and driving.

drug dependence Dalmane is not addictive in the same way as narcotics but, like other sedatives, it can be habit-forming to a certain extent if taken for a long period of time. If it is then stopped suddenly, some withdrawal symptoms may occur. There is a tendency toward physical and psychological dependency on the drug.

drug interactions Dalmane can increase the sedative effect of alcohol, antihistamines, other tranquilizers, and narcotics, sometimes to a dangerous extent. Unlike many sleeping pills, Dalmane does not interfere with the effect of the anticoagulant Coumadin.

see essays *Minor Tranquilizers. Sleeping Pills.*

Darvocet-N

generic ingredients

pain relievers =	propoxyphene, acetaminophen

Darvon

generic name

propoxyphene

Darvon Compound 65

generic ingredients

pain relievers =	propoxyphene, aspirin, phenacetin
mild stimulant =	caffeine

action and uses   Like aspirin, Darvon and its variants are used for the relief of mild to moderate pain. Unlike aspirin, however, Darvon's main ingredient, propoxyphene, cannot reduce fever and inflammation. The Darvon Compound 65 has the added pain relieving effects of the aspirin and phenacetin and Darvocet-N has the added pain reliever acetaminophen which can reduce fever but not inflammation. In recent years, the Darvon drugs have been among the most frequently prescribed in the United States. Though tests have shown that Darvon alone is usually no more effective in relieving pain than aspirin, and in some cases no more effective than a placebo (a pill with no active ingredient), there is a widespread belief that it is "stronger than aspirin." This may well be true of Darvon Compound and Darvocet-N, which include additional pain relievers. But psychological factors probably also play a role in the Darvon drugs' potent image. For one thing, Darvon and its variants can only be obtained on prescritpion, a fact which automatically suggests a special power. This impression is reinforced by their colorful packaging; a bright red tablet (such as Darvocet-N) or a pink and grey capsule (such as Darvon Compound 65) simply *looks* as though it would be more effective than two plain white aspirins. As is the case with many medications, the user's expectations of the drug can be an influential factor in determining its effectiveness.

adult dosage   Usually 32-65 mg (of propoxyphene) every 4 hours as needed for pain.

adverse effects   Side effects with Darvon alone are minimal, though some patients do experience nausea, dizziness, headache or allergic skin rashes. In the case of Darvon Compound 65 and Darvocet-N, their additional ingredients may cause additional side effects. The aspirin in Darvon Compound 65 can cause stomach irritation and bleeding if the drug is taken in large quantities or over an extended period. The phenacetin in Darvon Compound 65 can, if taken in large doses or over an extended period, cause kidney damage, while large doses of Darvon-N can cause liver damage.

precautions   Darvon Compound 65 should be used with caution by patients with stomach disorders or impaired kidney function and by pregnant or potentially pregnant women. Darvocet-N should be used with caution by patients with impaired liver function.

drug interactions   The propoxyphene in all Darvon drugs may cause increased sedation in combination with sedatives, sleeping pills, tranquilizers, alcohol, and drugs containing narcotics. Because it contains aspirin, Darvon Compound 65 can add to the effects of anticoagulants to increase risk of bleeding and cortisone-like drugs to increase risk of ulcer.

drug dependence

The propoxyphene these drugs contain is chemically related to the narcotic analgesics and both addiction and death through overdose have occurred. For this reason, the Darvon group of drugs have been placed under scrunity by the Food and Drug Administration, for possible restriction.

see essays

Drugs for the Relief of Pain and/or Inflammation. Non-Narcotic Pain Relievers.

Demerol

generic name

meperidine (available by generic name)

action and uses

A common narcotic pain reliever used by injection in hospital and occasionally taken orally. It is used in preoperative preparation for surgery, but is primarily used to relieve severe pain after surgery, and with other pain disorders such as cancer. It is available outside the hospital only with restricted prescriptions.

adult dosage

75-150 mg orally or by injection every 3-6 hours for pain.

adverse effects

A number of people experience nausea and vomiting when given this drug. This is not an allergy, but an increased sensitivity to one of its effects. It can also cause constipation, and in some, dizziness, or unusual sensations or dreams.

precautions

Demerol should only be used when other less potent pain relievers are not effective. It should be used with caution in persons with chronic lung disease or emphysema.

drug dependence

Tolerance and addiction to Demerol can and do occur with continued use, and withdrawal symptoms will occur when suddenly discontinued.

drug interactions

Demerol can add to the sedative and breathing depression effects of sedatives, tranquilizers and alcohol. It can also add to the constipating effects of many antispasmodic drugs and antihistamines.

see essay

Narcotic Pain Relievers.

Demulen-21

generic ingredients

progestogen = ethynodiol diacetate estrogen = ethinyl estradiol

action and uses

Demulen is one of many combination birth control pills containing a progesterone-like drug and an estrogen. It acts like most other oral contraceptives to prevent conception by affecting pituitary control of reproduction as well as acting locally on the lining of the uterus and the cervical mucus, and possibly in other ways. When taken regularly it is a very effective contraceptive drug. It is similar to Ovulen except for a somewhat lower amount and slightly different kind of estrogen.

adult dosage

In general, one tablet is taken daily (usually at night) on the first cycle, beginning on the 5th day of menstruation and continuing for 21 days. The pill is then discontinued for 7 days and restarted on the 8th day for another 21-day cycle.

adverse effects

Like all oral contraceptives, a variety of side effects may occur including weight gain, increased appetite, depression or fatigue, breast changes, gastrointestinal upset, headache, and increased vaginal discharge or infection. More significant but less common side effects include the risk of thrombophlebitis, increased blood pressure, increased blood sugar and gallbladder disease. The risk of certain side effects such as heart disease and gallbladder disease appear to increase with age (especially over the age of 35) while a history of true migraine headaches is associated with increased headaches and risk (though small) of actual strokes.

precautions

A history of thrombophlebitis, blood clots and migraine headaches is usually a relative contraindication to the usduse of oral contraceptives. For women with other risk factors, such as age over 35, history of heavy smoking, gallbladder disease, diabetes or high blood pressure, use should be weighed carefully against alternative birth control methods.

drug interactions

Several drug interactions have been suggested but none have been well-documented as significant in most cases.

see essays

Hormonal Drugs. Oral Contraceptives.

Diabinese

generic name

chlorpropamide

action and uses

A drug which lowers glucose levels in the blood, used to treat diabetes. Because Diabinese can be taken orally (unlike insulin) it is termed an "oral hypoglycemic" drug. It is similar to other oral antidiabetic drugs such as Orinase and Tolinase, but not DBI. Diabinese works by stimulating the pancreas to produce insulin and by helping the cells to use glucose. It is only of value in diabetics who are able to make insulin. Such patients usually have mild diabetes which often becomes evident toward middle age (and is therefore known as maturity onset diabetes). Oral hypoglycemic drugs should only be taken if dietary measures alone have failed to control the condition. Resistance to the effects of Diabinese often develops after a few months to years. It is recommended that withdrawal of oral antidiabetic drugs be tried every six months to one year since their continued use may not be needed. The long term benefits versus risks of this and related drugs are now widely debated.

adverse effects

The most common and hazardous adverse effect is excessive *lowering* of the blood sugar, which can cause symptoms of dizziness, weakness, cold sweats and mental dullness. Older persons and those on several other drugs (see drug interactions below) or with liver or kidney disease are more prone to this. In proper dosage, other side effects are unusual, but rashes, blood or liver abnormalities and water retention can occur.

adult dosage

This is individualized according to response. Initially 250 mg is given once daily and adjusted. Older patients may require lower doses.

precautions

The drug should be avoided by pregnant or potentially pregnant and nursing women as well as those with significant kidney, or liver diseases. Those allergic to sulfa drugs may develop an allergy to this drug.

drug interactions

Thiazide diuretics (such as hydrochlorothiazide, Diuril, Hygroton) can aggravate diabetes and may increase the dose requirement of the oral antidiabetic drug. A number of drugs can increase the risk of low blood sugar due to increased levels of drug. These include insulin, sulfa drugs, anti-inflammatory drugs such as aspirin, Butazolidin and Tandearil, and the anticonvulsant Dilantin. Inderal (prop-

153

ranolol) can also cause dangerous interactions and disguise the symptoms of hypoglycemia. Alcohol can cause a flushing reaction when taken with this drug.

see essay *Drugs for Diabetes.*

Diamox

generic name

acetazolamide (available by generic name)

action and uses A mild diuretic which promotes the loss of water from the body. It is used to treat glaucoma (caused by increased pressure of the fluid within the eye) and it also has a use in the treatment of epilepsy. Rarely it is used to treat other water retention states. Diamox acts by inhibiting an enzyme called carbonic anhydrase which is important for the excretion of excess acid by the kidney. When the enzyme is inhibited by the drug the kidney retains acid, but excretes more sodium and potassium and, as a result, more urine forms. The acid accumulated in the blood causes the drug to lose its effectiveness and the drug's action is only seen for a few days.

In glaucoma, the action is due to a local effect in the eye and although the same enzyme is acted upon by the drug, the same loss of the drug's activity does not occur. The action of Diamox in epilepsy is not fully understood, but inhibition of the enzyme carbonic anhydrase in the brain is thought to cut down the nervous discharges which lead to convulsions.

adult dosage Acetazolamide is supplied as tablets of 125 mg and 250 mg (Diamox), and as a sustained-release preparation (Sequels) of 500 mg. The dosage varies with the condition being treated, but is often one Sequel twice daily or one 250 mg Diamox tablet once to four times daily.

precautions Diamox is chemically related to the sulfa drugs, so if there is some allergy to this group of drugs, there may be allergy to Diamox as well. Diamox should be avoided by pregnant, potentially pregnant and nursing women.

adverse effects Tingling feelings in the fingers and toes may be experienced, and if taken for longer periods, weakness, drowsiness and dizziness may also occur.

drug interactions Diamox makes the urine alkaline and this can prevent the action of certain bladder antiseptics, and increase the action of certain drugs which are eliminated in the kidneys, such as quinidine, and Pronestyl.

see essays *Diuretics. Drugs for Seizures or Convulsions.*

Dicyclomine (generic name). See BENTYL.

Diethylpropion (generic name). See TENUATE.

Digoxin

trade names

Lanoxin, SK-Digoxin

action and uses
A drug used in treating heart failure. It increases the force of the heart muscle's contraction, slows the heart rate, and enables the heart to pump more efficiently. Like digitalis, of which it is a purer form, digoxin is derived from the foxglove plant, whose usefulness as a heart medicine was known to folk practitioners centuries before it was first written up by a British doctor in the late 1700s.

adult dosage
Dosage must be carefully adjusted according to individual responses and requirements. Usually, however, it is 0.125 mg to 0.25 mg taken once a day. It is sometimes given in a larger dose at first, but this has to be individually determined, often with careful checking of the pulse and an electrocardiogram, plus laboratory checks on blood levels of the drug.

adverse effects
For each patient, there is a very narrow margin between the amount of digoxin necessary to benefit the heart, and the amount liable to cause toxic effect. The symptoms of overdosage can include loss of appetite, nausea, vomiting, diarrhea, headache, blurred vision, and/or rapid, fluttering, irregular or skipped heartbeat.

precautions
Any of these symptoms should be reported to the doctor promptly. It cannot be overemphasized that this drug must only be taken under the strict supervision of a physician who can monitor its effect.

drug interactions
The diuretics ("water pills") often prescribed along with digoxin to treat excess fluid retention can increase the body's vulnerability to digoxin's toxic effects by causing excessive potassium loss. (Exceptions are the potassium-*retaining* diuretics Aldactazide, Aldactone, Diazide, and Dyranium). It may be necessary therefore, to supplement the body's potassium level daily with oral potassium preparations (KCl) or potassium-rich foods such as orange or tomato juice, bananas or dried fruit. The possibility of toxic effects with digoxin can also be increased by drugs for high blood pressure containing reserpine, by cortisone-like drugs such as prednisone, and by thyroid preparations.

see essay
Drugs for Heart Failure.

Dilantin

generic name

diphenylhydantoin or phenytoin (available by generic name)

action and uses

A drug used to prevent or reduce the frequency of epileptic seizures, which occur without apparent cause or are due to brain damage from accidents, surgery or strokes. If ineffective alone, it is given in combination with other anticonvulsant drugs such as phenobarbital. It is used rarely to treat irregular heart rhythms.

adult dosage

The usual dose is 300 mg orally once daily or in divided doses. The requirements vary widely so the need for dose adjustment is frequent when the drug is started.

adverse effects

The most common adverse effects are related to excess dosage and include unsteadiness in walking and difficulty in coordination, speech and bizarre behaviour or confusion. These effects will decrease with lower doses. Although Dilantin is usually well tolerated at proper doses, some may experience gastric upset, constipation, allergic skin rashes (which require stopping the drug), and swelling of the gums (often prevented by good dental hygiene and gum massage). Also, abnormalities of the blood cells and lymph glands can occur infrequently.

precautions

Dilantin should not be used in pregnancy unless the benefits outweigh the risks, since some studies have suggested this drug may harm the fetus.

drug interactions

Dilantin can interact with several drugs. When given with oral antidiabetic drugs, certain sulfa drugs, the anticoagulant Coumadin, the anti-inflammatory drug Butazolidin, and the anti-tuberculosis drug INH, the effects of Dilantin itself, as well as of these drugs, may be hazardously increased. Since some tricyclic antidepressants such as Elavil, and major tranquilizers such as Thorazine, increase the likelihood of seizures, they may decrease the effect of Dilantin and require an increased dose. Further, Dilantin may affect the metabolism of other drugs and decrease their effectiveness.

see essay

Drugs for Seizures or Convulsions.

Dimetane Expectorant

generic
ingredients

antihistamine = brompheniramine
decongestants = phenylephrine,
phenylpropanolamine
expectorant = guaifenesin

Dimetane Expectorant-DC

generic
ingredients

antihistamine = brompheniramine
decongestants = phenylephrine,
phenylpropanolamine
expectorant = guaifenesin
cough suppressant = codeine

action and uses
This is a compound mixture of cough/cold ingredients, aimed at several of the symptoms of a cold; it includes an antihistamine and decongestants for nasal congestion, and both an expectorant and, in the Dimetane Expectorant-DC, an antiussive for symptoms of cough. Whether all of these components can act effectively together is difficult to determine, but the inclusion of codeine, in the "DC" form, makes that mixture restricted for use when coughing might be harmful. If this is not the case, then the mixture without codeine is preferable.

adult dosage
The usual dose is one teaspoon or 5 ml of the syrup 3 to 4 times per day.

adverse effects
Side effects may include drowsiness due to the antihistamine and possibly palpitation due to the decongestants. Although the amount of codeine is small, it may cause nausea, and vomiting and if used for several days, may cause constipation. The expectorant may also cause nausea.

precautions
Driving or operating heavy equipment may be hazardous as sedation is an effect of this medication. Persons taking medicine for high blood pressure or heart ailments should check with their physicians before using, since the decongestants may elevate the blood pressure. Repeated use for any period more than 2-4 days is not desired in most cases. Dimetane should be avoided by pregnant and potentially pregnant and nursing women.

drug
dependence
The codeine in the "DC" compound can cause habituation if taken for prolonged periods.

drug interactions
The sedative effects of the antihistamine, and to a lesser

extent the codeine, can be additive to any other sedating drug such as tranquilizers and alcohol. The decongestants can raise the blood pressure and thus counteract the effect of any drug used to treat high blood pressure.

see essay *Drugs for Coughs and Colds*.

Dimetane

generic name

> brompheniramine (available by generic name)

action and uses A commonly prescribed antihistamine which is frequently used to treat allergic conditions, especially allergic rhinitis, sinusitis or conjunctivitis (redness of the eye). It shares the effects of most other antihistamines by blocking the effects of histamine and thus can decrease itching of the skin due to allergies, hives or rashes. It also can sometimes have a sedating effect, although it is not customarily used for this. It is not useful for treatment of asthma. It is usually much less expensive in generic form, as brompheniramine.

adult dosage Dimetane is available in oral tablets and liquid forms and for injections. The usual oral dose in 4 mg two to six times daily or one 8 mg or 12 mg Extentab twice daily as needed for treatment of allergic conditions.

adverse effects Although possibly less frequent than with some other antihistamines Dimetane may also cause significant sedation in some people. Other side effects are relatively rare, but can include dry mouth, blurred vision, or difficulty urinating, especially in older persons or those with glaucoma or prostate trouble.

drug interactions Dimetane is additive to other sedative or tranquilizing drugs and alcohol. It is also additive to other antispasmodic drugs used to treat ulcers or stomach problems, such as Pro-Banthine or Librax, to cause excessive dry mouth, constipation and difficulty in urinating.

precautions The sedative effects may interfere with driving or operating machinery. This drug should be used with caution in those with glaucoma or prostate trouble. It should also be avoided by pregnant or potentially pregnant women and nursing mothers.

see essay *Antihistamines*.

Dimetapp

| generic ingredients | antihistamine = brompheniramine
decongestants = phenylpropanolamine
phenylephrine |

action and uses   This mixture of an antihistamine and two decongestants is used for the usual symptoms of a cold: nasal congestion and a runny nose. It is one of many similar mixtures of decongestants and antihistamines sold for this purpose. It is also relatively effective for nasal congestion related to other causes such as allergies, but it is not useful in asthma.

adult dosage   Extentab: One tablet every 8-12 hours.

Elixir: 1-2 teaspoons, 3 or 4 times a day (the elixir has a slightly lower dose of the separate ingredients so it can be taken more frequently).

adverse effects   Side effects may include drowsiness due to the antihistamine and possibly palpitations due to the decongestants.

precautions   This drug should be avoided by pregnant, potentially pregnant and nursing women. Driving or operating heavy equipment may be hazardous if sedation is a side effect. Persons taking medicines for high blood pressure or heart ailments should check with their physicians before using Dimetapp since the decongestants may elevate the blood pressure.

drug interactions   The sedative effect of the antihistamine can add to other sedating drugs such as tranquilizers and alcohol. The decongestants can also raise the blood pressure and thus counteract the effect of any drug used to treat high blood pressure, such as Aldomet and Inderal.

see essay   *Drugs for Coughs and Colds.*

Diphenhydramine (generic name). See BENADRYL.

Diphenylhydantoin (generic name). See DILANTIN.

Diupres

| generic ingredients | antihypertensive = reserpine
diuretic = chlorothiazide |

action and uses   One of several popular fixed combination drugs prescribed for the control of high blood pressure. The reserpine in Diupres lowers blood pressure by blocking the sympathetic nervous system which constricts the blood vessels.

Diupres' other component, chlorothiazide, is a diuretic ("water pill"), which lowers blood pressure by promoting the elmination of excess salt and water from the system, thus decreasing blood volume and slightly dilating the blood vessels. Diupres is a fixed-dose combination drug – that is, it combines two ingredients in fixed amounts. This can be a drawback, because it limits the individualized dosage adjustment that is so often necessary with drugs for high blood pressure. If the amount of one of the ingredients in Diupres suits a patient, but the amount of the other does not, it may be simpler (and less expensive) for the patient to take the two drugs separately.

adult dosage
Usually 1-4 tablets per day if Diupres-250 has been prescribed, or 1-2 tablets per day if Diupres-500 has been prescribed.

Often it needs to be taken only once daily.

adverse effects
The reserpine in Diupres can cause drowsiness and lethargy, nasal stuffiness and stomach upset or ulceration, and sometimes, severe depression. The chlorothiazide in Diupres can cause allergic skin rash, nausea, diarrhea and excessive loss of potassium. This last-mentioned side effect may be signaled by muscle cramping and weakness, and can be corrected by eating potassium-rich foods (tomato and orange juice, bananas and dried fruit) or with a supplement of potassium chloride (KCl). Less frequently, chlorothiazide can precipitate gout or diabetes, possiblities which should be checked with blood tests at intervals.

precautions
Diupres should be used with caution by patients with gout or diabetes, a history of depression, heart failure, epilepsy, or peptic ulcers. It should be avoided if possible by pregnant or potentially pregnant women and nursing mothers. Women taking this drug for long periods of time should have regular breast checks.

drug interactions
Because of the reserpine it contains, Diupres can cause oversedation when taken concurrently with sedatives, sleeping pills, tranquilizers, antihistamines and alcohol. Some drugs for asthma, weight loss, depression, and colds can interact with reserpine to increase blood pressure. Diupres and any of these drugs, therefore, should not be taken concurrently except under a doctor's supervision. The chlorothiazide in Diupres can interact with steroids such as prednisone to cause excessive potassium loss. The increased potassium loss due to chlorothiazide can also increase sensitivity to the toxic effects of digoxin.

see essays
Drugs for High Blood Pressure. Diuretics.

Diuril

generic name

chlorothiazide (available by generic name)

action and uses

A diuretic ("water pill") used to treat high blood pressure and the excessive retention of water associated with certain heart, liver and kidney disorders and premenstrual tension. Its primary action is to cause a loss of excess salt and water via the kidneys, thus relieving edema (the swelling of body tissue due to fluid retention). It is also very useful in treating high blood pressure because it slightly relaxes the blood vessels and increases the effectiveness of other drugs used to lower blood pressure. This drug is a prototype of a group of diuretic drugs called *thiazide diuretics*. The terms "thiazide" refers both to a chemical structure and a class of several similar drugs, including Hydro-Diuril, Hygroton, Renese and Naturetin, which all share similar actions and side effects.

adult dosage

Usually 0.5 to 1.0 gram per day in divided doses of 250 or 500 mg. Increased urination occurs 1-2 hours after taking the drug and may last for 3-6 hours. Once the urination pattern is established the time at which the drug is taken can be determined for convenience. A night-time dose is usually impractical.

adverse effects

If taking Diuril causes the loss of too much of the essential mineral salt potassium, side effects may occur. These include weakness, tiredness, and dizziness. If potassium loss is very great it may be hazardous. Potassium supplements (KCl) are sometimes used in conjunction with Diuril. Potassium replacement can also be accomplished by dietary means (orange juice, tomato juice or bananas). Other side effects include a tendency to cause high blood sugar in individuals predisposed to diabetes. In some people Diuril can cause an elevation in blood uric acid levels (the substance in the blood which can cause gout). On long-term therapy these factors are checked but seldom cause a problem. Allergies to Diuril can occur but are not common.

precautions

This drug should be used with careful supervision, if at all, in pregnant or potentially pregnant women, and in persons with gout or diabetes.

drug interactions

Taken in conjunction with cortisone-like drugs, such as prednisone Diuril can cause excessive potassium loss. Potentially serious interactions may also occur if Diuril is taken in conjunction with digitalis drugs for the heart, because if and when too much potassium is eliminated from the system by the chlorothiazide, the heart can become sensitive to the toxic effects of digitalis. Medical supervision is essential.

see essays

Drugs for High Blood Pressure. Diuretics. Drugs for Heart Failure.

Donnagel-P.G.

generic
ingredients

```
antispasmodics = atropine,
                 hyoscine,
                 hyoscyamine
       narcotic = opium
 bulk producers = kaolin, pectin
```

action and uses

A mixture used to treat diarrhea. The exact cause of diarrhea is often never established. Donnagel-P.G., which treats the symptoms rather than the cause, reduces diarrhea in several ways. Kaolin and pectin provide bulk which reduce the looseness of the feces, and also bind with the irritant substances so that the latter leave the body along with the kaolin and pectin. The antispasmodic drugs atropine, hyoscine and hyoscyamine all reduce the actions of nerves which stimulate intestinal motion. The small dose of opium (equivalent to 6 ml of paregoric) relaxes the muscle of the intestine, relieving cramp and slowing intestinal movements. Although Donnagel-P.G. may be effective on a short-term basis, some authorities feel that prolonged use of this type of antidiarrheal may actually prolong the illness by allowing retention of the bacteria or toxins in the bowel.

adult dosage

Two tablespoons every three hours, as needed.

adverse
reactions

The anticholinergic-antispasmodics atropine, hyoscine and hyoscyamine can cause dry mouth, blurring of vision and difficulty in urination. If taken in excessive dose, it may cause vomiting, sedation, fever or flushing.

precautions

Persons with glaucoma or prostate trouble should take Donnagel-P.G. with caution. If diarrhea persists for more than a few days, the doctor should be consulted as the cause should be investigated.

drug
dependence

Opium is a narcotic, and though present in only small amounts can be habit-forming, another reason why Donnagel-P.G. should not be taken for more than a few days.

drug interactions	The antispasmodics and opium can have additive effects with other anticholinergic drugs such as antihistamines, cough/cold medicines and tricyclic antidepressants.
see essay	*Drugs for Diarrhea*.

Donnatal

generic
ingredients
	antispasmodics = atropine,
	                     hyoscine,
	                     hyoscyamine
	    tranquilizer = phenobarbital

action and uses	A fixed combination drug used to treat the symptoms of ulcers and intestinal disorders. The antispasmodics relax the smooth muscle of the stomach and small and large intestine and reduce spasm by acting on the nervous system. The phenobarbital is a sedative or anti-anxiety agent, added on the unproven assumption that decreasing anxiety will help relieve gastrointestinal symptoms. Donnatal is used to treat stomach and duodenal ulcers, irritable colon, spastic colon and intestinal upsets. Single antispasmodic drugs are likely to be as effective.
adult dosage	Usually one or two tablets, capsules or teaspoonfuls of liquid, three or four times per day. Donnatal No.2 contains twice as much phenobarbital as ordinary Donnatal. The dose must be adjusted to the individual needs of the patient, but is usually one or two tablets three times per day.
adverse effects	The primary side effects are due to the antispasmodics. These can include blurred vision, dryness of the mouth and skin and difficulty in urination, especially in older persons. They can also cause drying of bronchial secretions. Although the amount of phenobarbital present is small, it may cause sedation, and allergic reactions can occur.
precautions	Donnatal should be used with caution by persons with glaucoma, enlargement of the prostate, and chronic lung disease. If drowsiness occurs, driving or operating machinery may be hazardous.
drug dependence	Phenobarbital, one of the ingredients of Donnatal, is a barbiturate which may cause physical or psychological dependence if used over a long period.
drug interactions	The antispasmodics can have additive effects when taken with antihistamines, cough/cold medicines and tricyclic antidepressants, causing excessive dry mouth, constipation and occasional bladder problems. The

phenobarbital can decrease the effect of the anticoagulant, Coumadin, and might potentially add to the effects of other sedatives, tranquilizers or alcohol.

see essays   *Drugs for Nausea, Stomach Upset and Ulcers. Minor Tranquilizers.*

Doriden

generic name

glutethimide (available by generic name)

action and uses   A sleeping pill and sedative. Once the 6th most popular such drug in the United States, Doriden is now much less frequently prescribed because it is lethal when taken in overdose. Though still used as a night time sedative, it is gradually being replaced by newer and safer drugs. Doriden takes effect in about 30 minutes, and the sleep it induces lasts about 4-6 hours.

adult dosage   Usually 0.5 gram at bedtime.

adverse effects   In common with other sedatives and sleeping pills, Doriden can cause dizziness, headache and morning hangover. Allergic skin rashes are another possible side effect, as are changes in the blood cells which may result in weakness, fever, sore throat and bruises.

precautions   Doriden should not be taken by pregnant or potentially pregnant women, or by nursing mothers. It is necessary to exercise caution about driving or operating machinery when taking Doriden.

drug dependence   Doriden can produce both psychological and physical dependence. Occasionally, it causes withdrawal-like symptoms even while the drug is still being taken. When, after continuous use, the drug *is* stopped, the withdrawal symptoms can be severe.

drug interactions   The sedative effects of Doriden can be increased in combination with alcohol, tranquilizers, other sleeping pills and sedatives and antihistamines. Doriden can diminish the effect of anticoagulant drugs, such as Coumadin, thus increasing the chance of clotting.

see essay   *Sleeping Pills.*

Doxycycline (generic name). See VIBRAMYCIN.

Drixoral

generic ingredients	antihistamine = brompheniramine maleate decongestant = disoephedrine sulfate

action and uses A combination drug used to treat symptoms of colds and allergies. The antihistamine and decongestant help relieve nasal congestion and stop runny nose.

adult dosage The usual dose is one tablet or once or twice a day.

adverse effects Side effects may include drowsiness due to the antihistamine and possibly palpitation due to the decongestant.

precautions This drug should be avoided by pregnant, potentially pregnant or nursing women. Driving or operating heavy equipment may be hazardous if sedation is an effect of this medication. Those taking medicine for high blood pressure or heart ailments should check with their physicians before using, since the decongestant may elevate the blood pressure. Repeated use for any period more than two to four days is not desirable in most cases.

drug interactions The sedative effects of the antihistamine, can be additive to any other sedating drug such as tranquilizers and alcohol. The decongestant can raise the blood pressure and thus counteract the effect of any drug used to treat high blood pressure.

see essay *Drugs for Coughs and Colds.*

Dyazide

generic ingredients	diuretics = triamterene, hydrochlorothiazide

action and uses A fixed combination diuretic ("water pill") used in the treatment of high blood pressure and heart failure. Dyazide combines the action of two diuretics, one which retains potassium (triamterene) and one which causes loss of potassium (hydrochlorothiazide). Together they produce the desired loss of excess salt and water without the undesired effect of potassium loss. The fixed combination may present problems, however, since it does not allow dose adjustments of each of the individual ingredients. Increased urination usually occurs 1-2 hours after taking the drug.

adult dosage Usually one or two capsules once or twice a day.

adverse effects In some cases there may be a tendency to retain more potassium in the body than is needed or safe. When potassium levels rise too high there is a danger of heart failure and treatment to remove excess potassium is complex. This is not usually a problem, however, in persons with normal kidney function, but Dyazide can cause a decrease in kidney function, especially if there is pre-existing abnormal function. Dyazide can cause nausea or loss of appetite which can sometimes be associated with more serious abnormalities and require careful checking.

The hydrochlorothiazide in the drug may cause increased blood sugar in persons predisposed to diabetes. In some people it may cause an elevation in blood uric acid levels (the substance in the blood which can cause gout). Allergies to both of the drugs in Dyazide can occur.

precautions

Dyazide should not be used by pregnant or potentially pregnant women. Dyazide is not generally indicated in persons with any degree of kidney disease unless the blood is monitored for potassium and kidney function.

drug interactions

Preparations containing potassium can raise blood levels hazardously if given with Dyazide.

see essays

Drugs for High Blood Pressure. Diuretics. Drugs for Heart Failure.

E.E.S.

generic name

erythromycin ethyl succinate (available by generic name)

action and uses

A commonly used antibiotic which comes from the mold *Streptomyces*. It acts on bacteria to inhibit production of proteins but has no effect on human cells. E.E.S. (erythromycin) is most commonly used in mild to moderate infections where penicillin is indicated but allergy is present. These infections include bacterial sore throat ("strep throat"), respiratory or lung infections and some venereal diseases. It is seldom used in very serious infections.

adult dosage

The usual adult dosage is 250 to 500 mg every six hours, preferably on an empty stomach.

adverse effects

The most frequent side effect is gastrointestinal upset, including nausea, belching and diarrhea. Rashes and other allergic reactions can occur but are not as frequent as with other antibiotics.

precautions

This antibiotic like all others, should be taken for the time period directed, and every dose should be taken. Failure to do this can result in inadequate treatment of the infection, recurrence, or development of a resistant infection. E.E.S. should be used with caution by pregnant, potentially pregnant or nursing women.

drug interactions   Erythromycin may interfere with the effectiveness of penicillin and Cleocin.

see essay   *Drugs to Treat Infections.*

Elavil

generic name

amitriptyline

action and uses   A commonly-prescribed antidepressant drug. Like Tofranil and Sinequan, it belongs to a group of closely-related drugs called tricyclic antidepressants, and is used to treat certain types of moderately severe and longstanding depression. The tricyclic antidepressants are not true tranquilizers, although they can cause some sedation. Elavil's beneficial effect on mood and its ability to relieve depression are often quite marked, but there is usually a significant time-lag – before its antidepressant effects are felt.

adult dosage   The effective dose of Elavil is highly individualized and dosage adjustment may take one or two months. Initially, the dose is usually 25-75 mg per day, and may be increased to 150 mg per day. (The dose may be lower for elderly patients.) Because the drug is long-acting and may cause some sedation, it is usually taken just once a day, at bedtime.

adverse effects   Initially, Elavil may cause dry mouth, blurred vision, drowsiness, confusion or dizziness, constipation and difficulty in urination. (These effects are especially a problem in older people.) Other significant side effects may include effects on the heart rhythm.

precautions   Elavil should be taken with caution by persons with glaucoma, prostate gland problems, liver or heart disease, epilepsy, or with a hyperthyroid condition. It should not be used by pregnant or potentially pregnant or nursing women. It may interfere with driving or operating machinery.

drug interactions   Elavil can cause oversedation when taken in combination with alcohol, sleeping pills, tranquilizers, antihistamines, and drugs containing narcotics. It can add to the side effects of antispasmodic drugs and decrease the effects of drugs to lower blood pressure such as Ismclin. It can dangerously interfere with drugs to regulate heart rhythm, thyroid drugs, and drugs of the MAO inhibitor family (such as Marplan, Parnate and Nardil). Taken with drugs of the latter type, or with the sedative Placidyl, Elavil can cause delirium.

see essay   *Antidepressants.*

Elixophyllin

generic name

theophylline (available by generic name)

action and uses   Elixophyllin is both a capsule and liquid preparation of theophylline used to treat asthma. Theophylline is frequently the mainstay of the treatment of asthma and it can be prescribed as a less expensive generic form. It relaxes the smooth muscle constricting the small bronchi of the lungs and dilates the local arteries. The liquid form of Elixophyllin is rapidly absorbed and therefore rapidly effective. It is sometimes used for treatment of mild asthmatic attacks.

adult dosage   Capsule: One, 3-4 times daily.

Elixir: 1-2 teaspoons, 3-4 times daily. In general, the dose varies considerably from person to person and is adjusted on the basis of clinical response, change in lung function test, and/or blood level of the drug.

adverse effects   Most common side effect is gastric irritation from the direct effect of the drug in the stomach, as well as nausea and vomiting which is related to indirect effects of the theophylline. The nausea and vomiting may be decreased by lowering the dose. Other dose related effects also include headache, muscle cramps, palpitations and occasionally nervousness or insomnia.

precautions   Elixophyllin should be used with careful supervision in persons with irregular heart rhythms or other types of heart disease.

drug interactions   Elixophyllin is additive to other drugs used to treat asthma and side effects can also be additive. It is important for the prescribing physician to know all prescription and over-the-counter drugs used for treatment of this condition. Elixophyllin has effects on the clotting system which can alter the effects of blood-thinning drugs such as heparin or Coumadin.

see essay   *Drugs for Asthma and Lung Disease.*

Empirin Compound with Codeine

generic ingredients	narcotic pain reliever = codeine pain relievers = aspirin, phenacetin mild stimulant = caffeine

action and uses A combination drug used to treat moderate to severe pain. In addition to the ingredients found in Empirin Compound (the analgesics aspirin and phenacetin, plus the mild stimulant caffeine), this preparation contains the narcotic analgesic codeine, which makes the drug available on restricted prescription only.

adult dosage Usually 1-2 tablets every 3-6 hours as needed for pain.

adverse effects Like other combination pain relievers, the side effects of Empirin Compound with Codeine may include those of any of its ingredients, although the various components are present in lower doses than when used alone. Nonetheless, the aspirin present in Empirin Compound with Codeine can irritate the stomach, causing nausea, pain and even bleeding if taken in large quantities. The phenacetin in the preparation can, over a period of months, cause kidney damage, and the codeine can cause nausea, constipation, and drowsiness.

precautions Empirin Compound with Codeine should be avoided by patients with stomach disorders or impaired kidney function, and used with caution by pregnant or potentially pregnant or nursing mothers.

drug dependence Because of the codeine in this combination drug, habituation may occur if it is taken over a prolonged period of time.

drug interactions The aspirin in this combination drug can add to the effects of the anticoagulant Coumadin to increase risk of bleeding: taken in combination with cortisone-like drugs, it can increase the risk of a stomach ulceration. The codeine in the preparation can add to the sedative effects of alcohol, tranquilizers and antidepressants.

see essay *Narcotic Pain Relievers.*

E-Mycin

generic name	erythromycin (available by generic name)

action and uses A commonly used antibiotic which comes from the mold *Streptomyces*. It acts on bacteria to inhibit production of proteins but has no effect on human cells. Erythromycin is most commonly used in mild to moderate infections where penicillin is indicated but allergy is present. These infections include bacterial sore throat ("strep throat"), respiratory or lung infections and some venereal diseases. It is seldom used in very serious infections.

adult dosage The usual adult dosage is 250 to 500 mg every six hours, preferably on an empty stomach.

adverse effects The most frequent side effect is gastrointestinal upset, including nausea, belching and diarrhea. Rashes and other allergic reactions can occur but are not as frequent as with other antibiotics.

precautions This antibiotic, like all others, should be taken for the time period directed, and every dose should be taken. Failure to do this can result in inadequate treatment of the infection, recurrence, or development of a resistant infection. E-Mycin should be used with caution by pregnant, potentially pregnant and nursing women.

drug interactions Erythromycin may interfere with the effectiveness of penicillin and Cleocin.

see essay *Drugs to Treat Infections.*

Enduron

generic name

methyclothiazide

action and uses One of many types of diuretics or "water pills" of the thiazide type. Thus, it is very similar in its actions and side effects to hydrochlorothiazide, Esidrix, HyrdoDiuril and Diuril. It is used in the therapy of hypertension, heart failure and various other ailments where edema or swelling of the feet and/or hands is a problem. It acts by causing loss of water, sodium and potassium.

adult dosage 2.5 to 5 mg, once or twice daily.

adverse effects Like all thiazide diuretics, Enduron can cause excessive loss of potassium, which is seldom a problem at lower doses but can require potassium replacement at doses greater than 5 mg per day. This becomes more important if a person is taking digoxin or related drugs. Potassium can be replaced in the diet by orange and tomato juice and by bananas and dried fruit. Liquid potassium chloride (KCl) can also be taken. A significant lack of potassium can cause symptoms of weakness or dizziness or muscle cramp. In addition, Enduron can increase the blood sugar in acid and predispose to gout in some persons. It may also cause occasional allergic reactions.

precautions   Long-term use may require occasional checks of blood potassium, sugar and uric acid levels, especially if digitalis or digoxin is also taken. This drug should be used with caution by pregnant or potentially pregnant women.

drug interactions   The potassium loss caused by Enduron may predispose to toxicity of digitalis or digoxin. Since thiazide diuretics cause calcium retention, use of calcium-containing antacids, calcium supplements or vitamin D may cause elevated calcium in the blood. The potassium loss with steroid drugs (prednisone) can be additive to the effects of this drug.

see essays   *Drugs for High Blood Pressure. Drugs for Heart Failure. Diuretics.*

Equagesic

generic
ingredients

analgesics = aspirin ethoheptazine muscle relaxant = meprobamate

action and uses   A combination drug made up of two pain relievers and a muscle relaxant used to treat muscle pain and soreness. Interestingly enough, Equagesic's component drugs are present in lower doses than those usually thought necessary for effectiveness. For example, aspirin is usually taken in doses of 600 mg for relief of pain, but there is only 250 mg of aspirin in one Equagesic tablet. Similarly, meprobamate is usually administered in doses of 400-800 mg when used for its muscle-relaxant effect, but there is only 150 mg of meprobamate in one Equagesic tablet. The apparent explanation for the minimal presence of the components in Equagesic is that they are additive to one another's effects. But whether they are truly additive or effective at these low doses, is not completely clear. It is probable that an adequate dose of aspirin and the application of heat will often be as effective in treating sore muscles as this more expensive drug.

adult dosage   Usually 2 tablets 3-4 times daily.

adverse effects   As with other combination drugs, Equagesic has the side effects of its various components. The aspirin in Equagesic can irritate the stomach, causing nausea, vomiting, pain and bleeding. The ethoheptazine in Equagesic can cause dizziness and drowsiness. The meprobamate in Equagesic can cause headache, blurred vision, stomach upset, and allergic skin rashes.

precautions

Because of the meprobamate it contains, Equagesic should not be taken by pregnant or potentially pregnant women or nursing mothers. Because of the aspirin in Equagesic, it should be taken with caution by patients who have stomach disorders or a sensitivity to aspirin. It should not be used by persons taking Coumadin.

drug dependence

Because of the meprobamate it contains, Equagesic can, if taken in large doses over an extended period, cause psychological and/or physical dependence.

drug interactions

The aspirin in Equagesic can add to the effects of anticoagulants such as Coumadin and increase the risk of bleeding. The meprobamate in Equagesic can increase sedative effects of alcohol, tranquilizers, sleeping pills, and antidepressants, and counteract the effects of the anticoagulant Coumadin.

see essay

Non-Narcotic Pain Relievers.

Equanil

generic name

meprobamate (available by generic name)

action and uses

A minor tranquilizer used to relieve mild tension and anxiety. Both Equanil and Miltown (another trade name for meprobamate) are very similar to barbiturates in their sedative effects. Their use as sedatives, however, has diminished somewhat since the introduction of Librium and Valium. Equanil is also frequently used in cases of muscle strain (as in back strain) as a muscle relaxant. Whether its beneficial effect in such cases is due to sedation or to true muscle relaxation is not clear.

adult dosage

Usually 200-400 mg four times a day and sometimes double that dose.

adverse effects

The incidence of allergic reactions to Equanil is significant. Such reactions may include skin rashes or hives. Other common side effects may include nausea, headache, dizziness and excessive drowsiness.

precautions

Equanil should not be taken by pregnant, potentially pregnant or nursing women. It may interfere with driving or operating machinery.

drug dependence

Equanil can produce psychological and or physical dependence. Once habituation to the drug has developed, convulsions can occur if the drug is suddenly stopped, especially if the daily dose has been more than 800 mg four times a day.

drug interactions   Equanil's sedative effects can be increased by alcohol, other sedatives and tranquilizers, sleeping pills and antidepressants. Equanil can decrease the effects of anticoagulants, oral contraceptives, and the estrogens used in hormone replacement therapy, because it affects the way the liver metabolizes these drugs.

see essay   *Minor Tranquilizers.*

Erythrocin

generic name

erythromycin ethyl succinate (available by generic name)

The antibiotic is a form of erythromycin and shares its effects and adverse reactions as discussed below.

Erythromycin

trade names

E-Mycin, E.E.S., Erythrocin, Pediamycin, Ilotycin, Robimycin

action and uses   A commonly used antibiotic which comes from the mold *Streptomyces*. It acts on bacteria to inhibit production of proteins but has no effect on human cells. Erythromycin is most commonly used in mild to moderate infections where penicillin is indicated but allergy is present. These infections include bacterial sore throat (''strep throat''), respiratory or lung infections and some venereal diseases. It is seldom used in very serious infections.

adult dosage   The usual adult dosage is 250 to 500 mg every six hours, preferably on an empty stomach.

adverse effects   The most frequent side effect is gastointestinal upset, including nausea, belching and diarrhea. Rashes and other allergic reactions can occur but are not as frequent as with other antibiotics.

precautions   This antibiotic, like all others, should be taken for the time period directed, and every dose should be taken. Failure to do this can result in inadequate treatment of the infection, recurrence, or development of a resistant infection. Erythromycin should be used with caution by pregnant, potentially pregnant and nursing women.

drug interactions   Erythromycin may interfere with the effectiveness of penicillin and Cleocin.

see essay   *Drugs to Treat Infections.*

Esidrex (brand name for hydrochlorothiazide).
See HYDROCHLOROTHIAZIDE.

Etrafon

generic
ingredients

antidepressant = amitriptyline
major tranquilizer = perphenazine

action and uses

A combination drug promoted and used to treat moderate
to severe anxiety with depression. Etrafon contains two
potent drugs: amitriptyline, a tricyclic antidepressant used
in the treatment of moderate to severe depression; and
perphenazine, an antipyschotic drug, or major tranquilizer,
used in the treatment of psychoses, or thought disorders.
There is some question among medical authorities as to the
rationale behind the use of these two drugs in a fixed
combination form.

In the first place, both drugs when used alone require
careful, individualized dosage adjustment, something
which cannot be done with any subtlety when they are
combined. (Raising or lowering the dose of one drug in a
fixed combination automatically alters the dose of the
other as well.) Secondly, the adverse effects of the two
drugs are very similar and can be additive. Thirdly,
although Etrafon is promoted for the treatment of anxiety
with depression, neither of its two components is a true
anti-anxiety drug. One rationale for the use of this
combination drug is that the antidepressant amitriptyline
will on occasion produce a thought disorder which can be
suppressed by perphenazine, but whether this is true has
not been carefully established in clinical testing.

In the final analysis, it is questionable whether, in veiw
of their additive side effects, the use of these two potent
drugs is justified in any but truly serious mental disorders,
and then it is possible that only one is truly indicated.

adult dosage

Etrafon is available in four tablet sizes, which are
recommended 3-4 times per day, although since both
ingredients are very long acting they can usually be taken
once daily, usually in the evening to use the sedative
effect.

adverse effects

Etrafon has the combined side effects of its two
components, which in this case are significant and additive. Amitriptyline and perphenazine can both cause dry
mouth, blurred vision, urine retention, constipation, and
rapid or irregular heartbeat. Perphenazine can also cause

Parkinsonian symptoms (a rigid facial expression, stiff gait, and trembling in the hands, arms and feet), as well as dizziness, jaundice, blood disorders and severe skin rashes.

precautions
Etrafon should not be used by pregnant, potentially pregnant or nursing women.

Etrafon should be used with caution by patients with glaucoma, prostate gland trouble, heart disease, epilepsy, impaired liver function, or hyperthyroidism.

drug interactions
Oversedation is possible when Etrafon is combined with alcohol, other tranquilizers and antidepressants, sleeping pills, sedatives, and drugs containing narcotics. The amitriptyline in Etrafon can interfere with drugs to lower blood pressure, thyroid drugs, and drugs of the MAO inhibitor family (such as Marplan, Parnate and Nardil). The perphenazine in Etrafon can also interfere with drugs to lower blood pressure. Both drugs can be additive to antispasmodics and anti-Parkinsonian drugs to cause constipation.

see essay
Major Tranquilizers and Antidepressants.

Feosol

generic name

ferrous sulfate (available by generic name)

action and uses
A dietary supplement of iron used for treating anemia which results from iron deficiency. Iron is an important part of the protein hemoglobin, which is responsible for carrying oxygen in the red blood cells. If there is insufficient hemoglobin, not enough oxygen will reach the tissues of the body. Iron deficiency may be due to lack of iron in the diet or increased demand, as in pregnancy, failure of the body to absorb iron from the diet, or severe or chronic bleeding. Women lose iron due to blood loss during menstruation. In pregnancy iron is transferred from the mother to the developing child. Women therefore need more iron than men and this can be provided by a dietary supplement, though a well-rounded diet usually provides adequate iron without need for pills. Men almost never need iron supplements, except when prescribed by a doctor.

adult dosage
Usually 1 tablet or 2 teaspoonfuls 3 or 4 times per day, taken before meals.

adverse effects
Iron preparations can cause vomiting, abdominal cramp-

ing, and diarrhea, although this is not usually severe. Long-term use may lead to constipation. Feosol and other iron preparations will tend to produce black bowel movements. Prolonged use of unneeded iron can cause harmful iron deposits in the liver and heart.

precautions   If iron supplements are really needed in addition to the iron in the diet, they should be prescribed by a doctor.

drug interactions   Certain drugs can form complexes with iron to prevent its absorbtion from the intestine. These include tetracycline and antacids.

see essay   *Vitamins and Minerals*.

Ferrous sulfate (generic name). See FEOSOL.

Fiorinal

generic
ingredients

> pain relievers = aspirin, phenacetin
> minor tranquilizer = butalbital
> mild stimulant = caffeine

Fiorinal with Codeine

generic
ingredients

> narcotic pain reliever = codeine
> pain relievers = aspirin,
>   phenacetin
> minor tranquilizer = butalbital
> mild stimulant = caffeine

action and uses   Both of these combination drugs are prescribed for the relief of mild to moderate pain, particularly tension headache pain. Both are typical of the many drugs which add a sedative, tranquilizer or anti-anxiety drug (in this case, butalbital) to a drug or drugs aimed at relieving the actual problem (in this case, the pain relievers aspirin, phenacetin and codeine). In many cases, relief of the headache or other problem will in itself relieve the accompanying anxiety, so whether the addition of a sedative is useful, effective or worth the extra cost is somewhat doubtful. As for the inclusion of caffeine, the sum effect of a stimulant plus a sedative on tension or anxiety is equally unclear and unproven.

adult dosage   Usually 2 tablets every 3-6 hours as needed.

adverse effects   As with other combination drugs, Fiorinal and Fiorinal with Codeine have all the side effects of their various components. The aspirin they contain can cause severe stomach irritation and bleeding. The phenacetin can, over extended periods, cause kidney damage. The butalbital in both preparations can cause dizziness, headache or allergic reactions. Finally, the codeine in Fiorinal with Codeine can cause nausea and constipation.

precautions
Fiorinal and Fiorinal with Codeine should both be used with caution by patients with stomach disorders or impaired kidney function, those taking the anticoagulant Coumadin, and should be avoided by pregnant, potentially pregnant and nursing women.

drug dependence
The bultalbital in both preparations and the codeine in Fiorinal with Codeine can both cause psychological and or physical dependence if taken over extended periods.

drug interactions
The aspirin in both these preparations can add to the effect of anticoagulants, to increase hazard of bleeding, and with cortisone-like drugs and other anti-inflammatory drugs to increase the risk of ulcer. The butalbital in both preparations, and the codeine in Fiorinal with Codeine, can add to the sedative effect of other pain relievers, sleeping pills, tranquilizers, antidepressants, sedatives, alcohol and antihistamines. The butalbital can decrease the effect of the anticoagulant Coumadin.

see essays
Narcotic Pain Relievers. Non-Narcotic Pain Relievers.

Flagyl

generic name

> metronidazole

action and uses
The drug of choice used to treat vaginal infections due to the parasite Trichomonas, as well as certain other types of parasite infections, especially amebiasis. Vaginal infections due to Trichomonas are extremely common and usually cause a white foamy, itching discharge. A chronic infection can sometimes cause inflammation of the cervix and changes in the Pap smear, which is one important reason for treatment if an infection persists. Since the infection is transmitted by sexual contact, both partners are usually treated to prevent reinfection. Flagyl was once available as a local suppository, but this form of treatment was found to be generally ineffective. Until recently, the drug was used routinely on discovery of any Trichomonas, but because of concern for one potential side effect, described below, local treatment, including use of cotton underwear

and acid douche, is often tried before routine use.

adult dosage

For treatment of vaginal infections, the usual dose is 250 mg orally three times a day for seven days. More recently, it has been found that a single dose of 2000 mg (8 tablets) is effective in many cases, so this may also be suggested. The dose for other parasite infections is usually higher and individualized.

adverse effects

In general, serious side effects are unusual but certain bothersome side effects are common. Nausea, loss of appetite or gastric upset, as well as a metallic taste or furry tongue may be experienced. Less commonly, dizziness, headache, vertigo or burning on urination may occur. Flagyl may cause a temporary fall in the white blood count. There is concern that the ability of this drug to cause increased numbers of tumors in rats and mice may have significance in humans, but as yet, this relationship has not been shown in humans.

precautions

Alcohol should be avoided while taking this drug since reactions may occur. This drug should not be taken by pregnant or potentially pregnant women or nursing mothers nor in the presence of neurological disorders.

drug interactions

When Flagyl and alcohol are taken together, a certain number of people will experience marked nausea, vomiting, flushing, headaches and faintness. Flagyl can also interact with Antabuse, a drug used to treat alcoholism, to cause unpleasant reactions, including mental changes and confusion.

see essay

Drugs for Skin and Local Disorders.

Flurandrenolide (generic name). See CORDRAN.

Gantanol

generic name

sulfamethoxazole (available by generic name)

action and uses

A sulfonamide or "sulfa" drug. Gantanol is not an antibiotic but it prevents the growth of bacteria and is therefore used to treat some infections. It is particularly effective against infections of the kidney, bladder and urinary tract, including cystitis. Occasionally it is used to treat meningitis.

adult dosage

The initial dose is usually 2 grams, followed by 1 gram three times a day.

adverse effects

This drug may sometimes cause nausea, vomiting or

other gastrointestinal symptoms as well as headache or dizziness. Like all sulfa drugs, Gantanol may cause allergic reactions such as rashes, as well as very serious, life-threatening reactions with fever, severe rash, and kidney failure.

precautions It is always important to drink plenty of water while taking this drug to prevent crystal formation in the kidney. If any fever, nausea or rash occurs after starting the drug, it should be discontinued and the doctor notified. It should be avoided in persons with severe kidney disease and those with G6PD deficiency (a red blood cell disease). As in the treatment of all infections, it is important to take the drug for the full time recommended to prevent recurrence of the infection. Pregnant, potentially pregnant and nursing women should avoid this drug.

drug interactions As with many sulfa drugs, Gantanol may increase the effect of oral antidiabetic drugs (to cause low blood sugar) and Dilantin, Butazolidin, and phenobarbital to increase the likelihood of toxicity to these drugs.

see essay *Drugs to Treat Infections.*

Gantrisin

generic name

sulfisoxazole (available by generic name)

action and uses A sulfonamide or "sulfa" drug. Gantrisin is not an antibiotic but it prevents the growth of bacteria and is therefore used to treat some infections. It is particularly effective against infections of the kidney, bladder and urinary tract, including cystitis. Occasionally it is used to treat meningitis.

adult dosage Usually 2 to 4 grams initially, followed by 4 to 8 grams per day divided into at least four doses.

adverse effects This drug may sometimes cause nausea, vomiting or other gastrointestinal symptoms as well as headaches or dizziness. Like all sulfa drugs, Gantrisin may cause allergic reactions such as rashes, as well as very serious, life-threatening reactions with fever, severe rash, and kidney failure.

precautions It is always important to drink plenty of water while taking this drug to prevent crystal formation in the kidney. If any fever, nausea or rash occurs after starting the drug, it should be discontinued and the doctor notified. It should be avoided in persons with severe kidney disease and

G6PD deficiency (a red blood cell disease). As in the treatment of all infections, it is important to take the drug for the full time recommended to prevent recurrence of the infection. Pregnant, potentially pregnant and nursing women should avoid this drug if possible.

drug interactions As with many sulfa drugs, Gantrisin may increase the effect of oral antidiabetic drugs (to cause low blood sugar), and Dilantin, Butazolidin, and phenobarbital to increase the likelihood of toxicity to these drugs.

see essay *Drugs to Treat Infections.*

Glutethimide (generic name). See DORIDEN.

Hydergine

generic name

dihydroergotoxine

action and uses This drug generally relaxes blood vessels and as a result increases blood flow. Its main use now is to treat certain mental and emotional problems of the elderly which are thought to arise from a reduced blood flow to the brain. Infrequently it is used to treat conditions where there is not enough blood flowing through peripheral vessels. It has also been used to lower high blood pressure. It has been shown to be effective in elderly confused patients only when they also had elevated blood pressure.

adult dosage Hydergine is available as subligual tablets containing 0.5 mg or 1.0 mg of the combined active drugs. These tablets are not to be swallowed but must be allowed to dissolve slowly under the tongue. The recommended dose is 1 mg three times a day.

adverse effects These include nausea and vomiting, blurred vision, skin rashes and nasal stuffiness.

precautions Excessive dosing may constrict some blood vessels and limit blood flow to the extremities. This drug should not be taken by pregnant or potentially pregnant women.

drug interactions Hydergine may be additive to the effects of some drugs used for high blood pressures.

see essay *Drugs Used to Prevent or Treat Circulatory Problems.*

Hydralazine (generic name). See APRESOLINE.

Hydrochlorothiazide

trade names

Esidrex, HydroDiuril, Oretic

action and uses

The prototype diuretic ("water pill") used to treat high blood pressure and the excessive retention of water associated with certain heart, liver and kidney disorders and premenstrual tension. Its primary action is to cause a loss of excess salt and water via the kidneys, thus relieving edema (swelling of body tissue due to fluid retention). It is also very useful in treating high blood pressure because it slightly relaxes the blood vessels and increases the effectiveness of other drugs used to lower blood pressure. This drug is a prototype of a group of diuretic drugs called *thiazide diuretics*. The term "thiazide" refers both to a chemical structure and a class of several similar drugs, including Diuril, Hygroton, Renese and Naturetin, which all share similar actions and side effects.

adult dosage

Usually 50-100 mg per day (and sometimes 200 mg per day) in divided doses if more than 50 mg is taken. Hydrochlorothiazide usually takes effect within two hours and remains effective for 3-6 hours thereafter. During this period there may be a need to urinate frequently as the kidneys eliminate the body's excess fluid.

adverse effects

A dose of 50 mg per day of hydrochlorothiazide is rarely accompanied by side effects, but with long-term use and at higher doses, certain side effects may occur. Chief among these is the loss of the essential mineral potassium, which is eliminated from the body along with the excess salt and water. Symptoms of a significant drop in the body's natural potassium level may include dizziness, unusual tiredness, muscle cramps and/or tingling in the extremities. Fortunately, it is easy to replace lost potassium – by adding potassium rich foods (orange and tomato juice, dried fruits and bananas) to the diet; by using salt substitutes (Co-salt or Lite-salt); or with a supplement of potassium chloride (KCl). The amount of loss and need for potassium replacement is usually evaluated early in therapy by checking blood levels of potassium at intervals. Other side effects with hydrochlorothiazide may include an elevation of the blood sugar level in people predisposed to diabetes, and a rise in the body's uric acid level, which can precipitate gout. Both of these effects can be watched for, and rarely produce problems. Finally, some people are allergic to hydrochlorothiazide, developing reactive skin rashes or nausea; this is slightly more likely in people who are allergic to sulfa drugs or oral antidiabetic drugs.

precautions   This drug should be used with caution by pregnant or potentially pregnant or nursing women, and by patients with gout or diabetes.

drug interactions   Taken in conjunction with cortisone-like drugs such as prednisone, hydrochlorothiazide can cause excessive potassium loss. Potentially serious interactions may also occur if hydrochlorothiazide is taken in conjunction with digitalis drugs for the heart, because if and when too much potassium is eliminated from the system by the hydrochlorothiazide, the heart can become sensitive to the toxic effects of digitalis. Medical supervision is essential.

see essays   *Drugs for High Blood Pressure. Diuretics.*

HydroDiuril (brand name for hydrochlorothiazide). See HYDROCHLOROTHIAZIDE.

Hydropres

generic ingredients

antihypertensive drug = reserpine
diuretic = hydrochlorothiazide

action and uses   One of several popular fixed combination drugs prescribed for the control of high blood pressure. The reserpine in Hydropres lowers blood pressure by blocking the sympathetic nervous system which constricts the blood vessels. Hydropres' other component, hydrochlorothiazide, is a diuretic ("water pill"). It lowers blood pressure by promoting the elimination of excess salt and water from the system, thus decreasing blood volume and slightly dilating the blood vessels. Hydropres is a fixed-dose combination drug – that is, it combines two ingredients in fixed amounts. This can be a drawback, because it limits the individualized dosage adjustment that is so often necessary with drugs for high blood pressure. If the amount of one of the ingredients in Hydropres suits a patient, but the amount of the other does not, it may be simpler (and less expensive) for the patient to take the two drugs separately.

adult dosage   Usually 1-4 tablets per day if Hydropres-25 has been prescribed, or 1-2 tablets per day if Hydropres-50 has been prescribed. It often can be taken only once daily.

adverse effects   The reserpine in Hydropres can cause drowsiness and lethargy, nasal stuffiness and stomach upset or ulceration, and sometimes severe depression. The hydrochlorothiazide in Hydropres can cause allergic skin rash, nausea, diarrhea, and excessive potassium loss. This last-mentioned side effect may be signaled by muscle cramping and weakness, and can be corrected by eating potassium-rich foods (tomato and orange juice, bananas and dried fruit) or with a supplement of potassium chloride (KCl). Less frequently, hydrochlorothiazide can precipitate gout or diabetes, possibilities which should be checked with blood tests at intervals.

precautions

Hydropres should be used with caution by patients with gout or diabetes, a history of depression, heart failure, epilepsy, or peptic ulcers. It should be avoided if possible by pregnant or potentially pregnant women and nursing mothers.

drug interactions

Because of the reserpine it contains, Hydropres can cause oversedation when taken concurrently with sedatives, sleeping pills, tranquilizers, antihistamines and alcohol. Some drugs for asthma, weight loss, depression and colds can interact with reserpine to increase blood pressure. Hydropres and any of these drugs, therefore, should be used concurrently only under a doctor's supervision. The hydrochlorothiazide in Diupres can interact with steroids such as prednisone to cause excessive potassium loss. The increased potassium loss due to hydrochlorothiazide can also increase sensitivity to the toxic effects of digoxin.

see essays

Drugs for High Blood Pressure. Diuretics.

Hygroton

generic name

chlorthalidone

action and uses

A diuretic ("water pill") used to treat high blood pressure and the excessive retention of water associated with certain heart, liver and kidney disorders and premenstrual tension. Its primary action is to cause a loss of excess salt and water via the kidneys, thus relieving edema (the swelling of body tissue due to fluid retention). It is also very useful in treating high blood pressure because it slightly relaxes the blood vessels and increases the effectiveness of other drugs used to lower blood pressure. This drug is one of a group of diuretic drugs called *thiazide diuretics*. The term "thiazide" refers both to a chemical structure and a class of several similar drugs, including Diuril, Renese and Naturetin, which all share similar actions and side effects.

adult dosage

Usually 50-100 mg per day, although in some cases it can be taken on alternate days or less frequently, since it has a slightly greater effect than the same dose of hydrochlorothiazide. Increased urination occurs 3-12 hours or longer after taking the drug and once this is determined, a convenient time for dosing can be decided.

adverse effects

Hygroton can cause excessive loss of potassium, especially when taken daily. If this occurs potassium can be replaced either in the diet (extra orange juice, tomato juice, or bananas) or with liquid potassium chloride (KCl). Hygroton also tends to cause an increased blood sugar in those predisposed to diabetes and may increase uric acid levels (the substance in the blood which can cause gout). If used to excess, Hygroton or any diuretic can cause dehydration and may affect kidney function and the amount of waste products in the blood. The effects of the initial use of Hygroton are therefore usually followed carefully.

precautions

This drug should be used with caution by pregnant or potentially pregnant women, and by patients with gout or diabetes.

drug interactions

Taken in conjunction with cortisone-like drugs, such as prednisone, it can cause excessive potassium loss. Potentially serious interactions may also occur if Hygroton is taken in conjunction with digitalis drugs for the heart, because if and when too much potassium is eliminated from the system by the Hygroton, the heart can become sensitive to the toxic effects of digitalis. Medical supervision is essential.

see essays

Diuretics. Drugs for High Blood Pressure.

Ilosone

generic name

erythromycin estolate (available by generic name)

action and uses

A commonly used antibiotic which comes from the mold *Streptomyces*. It acts on bacteria to inhibit production of proteins but has no effect on human cells. Erythromycin is most commonly used in mild to moderate infections where penicillin is indicated but allergy is present. These infections include bacterial sore throat ("strep throat"), respiratory or lung infections and some venereal diseases. It is seldom used in very serious infections. Ilosone, unlike other erythromycins, is not as easily destroyed by stomach acid which gives more flexibility, in time of dosing, but this may not be worth the extra cost or risk of this special form.

adult dosage   The usual adult dosage is 250 to 500 mg every six hours.

adverse effects   The most frequent side effect is gastrointestinal upset, including nausea, belching and diarrhea. Rashes and other allergic reactions can occur but are not as frequent as with another antibiotics. Ilosone, unlike other erythromycin preparations, can have an allergic effect on the liver producing a yellowing of the skin and eyes, known as jaundice. This effect is rare and usually only appears if Ilosone is taken for more than ten days. It is preceeded by nausea, vomiting, pain in the abdomen and loss of energy. These symptoms disappear when the drug is discontinued.

precautions   This antibiotic, like all others, should be taken for the time period directed, and every dose should be taken. Failure to do this can result in inadequate treatment of the infection, recurrence, or development of a resistant infection. If the symptoms of adverse effects occur, such as abdominal pain, the doctor should be consulted promptly. Ilosone should be used with caution by pregnant, potentially pregnant and nursing women.

drug interactions   Erthromycin may interfere with the effectiveness of penicillin and Cleocin.

see essay   *Drugs to Treat Infections.*

Imipramine (generic name). See TO FRANIL.

Inderal

generic name

propranolol

action and uses   A drug used to treat high blood pressure, angina pectoris and certain types of irregular heart rhythm. The exact mechanism by which it lowers blood pressure in is not known, although it does block part of the sympathetic nervous system, which is responsible for constricting the blood vessels, and it does decrease both heart rate and the force of heart contraction, thus saving work for the heart. In the treatment of high blood pressure, Inderal is often used in conjunction with a diuretic ("water pill") such as hydrochlorothiazide, and or a drug to dilate blood vessels, such as Apresoline.

adult dosage   Initially, usually 10-20 mg, 3-4 times per day, with a gradual increase until the desired blood pressure response is achieved. The usual effective dosage range is 120-320 mg daily in divided doses, usually taken before meals and at bedtime. It is normally recommended that if Inderal is to be discontinued, the drug should be stopped gradually, over a period of days or weeks.

adverse effects   The major side effects of Inderal tend to occur early in therapy and include dizziness, slow heart rate, tiredness and depression, increased dreaming, gastrointestinal upset, skin rashes, cold hands and feet, and increased wheezing in patients who have asthma, or chronic lung disease.

precautions   Inderal should be used with caution by pregnant or potentially pregnant women. It should be avoided by those with asthma, diabetes and in most cases of definite heart failure, except when the heart failure is caused by high blood pressure, or certain irregular heart rhythms.

drug interactions   Inderal may interact harmfully with insulin and antidiabetic drugs, and with MAO inhibitor drugs such as the antidepressants Marplan, Nardil and Parnate, the antibiotic Furoxine and the drug Tegretol. Inderal can usefully add to the effects of drugs for high blood pressure but interact harmfully to increase the blood pressure with nasal decongestants like Neosynephrine and cough/cold preparations. With reserpine, barbiturates and narcotics, Inderal may cause oversedation.

see essays   *Drugs for High Blood Pressure. Diuretics. Drugs for Angina Pectoris. Drugs for Abnormal Heart Rhythms.*

Indocin

generic name

> indomethacin

action and uses   Indocin is one of several drugs used as an alternative to aspirin in the treatment of various types of arthritis. It has the ability to relieve pain and decrease inflammation associated with arthritis, but it has no effect on the progress of the disease. Indocin was released over 10 years ago as a potential alternative to aspirin and received wide use. However, the occurrence of the various side effects resulted in decreased and more selective use. It is one of several anti-inflammatory drugs, such as Motrin, Naprosyn, Nalfon and Tolectin, which serve as alternatives in arthritis therapy when an adequate trial of aspirin has not been successful or tolerated.

adult dosage 25 mg, 2 or 3 times a day with gradual increases of dose according to response up to a daily dose of 150 to 200 mg.

adverse effects The most common side effects are due to irritation of the gastrointestinal tract which can include ulceration and bleeding. In addition, visual changes, hearing changes, headache, edema and dizziness may occur. Rarely, abnormalities of the blood and liver have been observed.

precautions Indocin should not be used by pregnant, potentially pregnant or nursing women. It is not advised for people with known ulcer disease or allergy to aspirin. If taken for long periods, periodic eye examinations are indicated. Occasionally Indocin may cause sufficient drowsiness to interfere with driving or operating machinery. The prescribing physician should be notified if any symptoms of headache, visual or hearing changes or personality changes occur.

drug interactions Indocin may increase the likelihood of bleeding when used with oral anticoagulants such as Coumadin. The likelihood of peptic ulcer is also increased when used with other drugs predisposing to ulcer such as prednisone or aspirin.

see essay *Drugs for Pain with Inflammation.*

Ionamin

generic name

phentermine (available by generic name)

action and uses An appetitie suppressant used as an aid in weight reduction. Its effect in decreasing the appetite tends to diminish after 7-14 days. Its true effectiveness in causing weight loss can be questioned. Like amphetamine sulfate, to which it is related, it also stimulates the nervous system, producing an increase in energy and mental alertness and a lift in mood. Though Ionamine is less effective in suppressing appetite than amphetamine sulfate, it is probably preferable because it may have less tendency to cause dependence.

adult dosage Usually 25 mg before meals, 3 times daily.

adverse effects Like amphetamine sulfate, Ionamin can cause dry mouth, nervousness, headache, anxiety, nausea, vomiting, rapid, irregular heartbeat and elevation of the blood

187

pressure. (In most patients, however, the side effects of Ionamin on the nervous system and cardiovascular system are less marked than they are with amphetamine sulfate). Withdrawal symptoms of fatigue and depression are likely when the drug is stopped, particularly if it has been taken in doses exceeding those prescribed.

precautions
Ionamin should only be used for short periods under careful supervision. It should not be used by anyone with any type of heart disease or irregular heart rhythm or high blood pressure.

drug dependence
As with amphetamine sulfate, Ionamin can cause severe psychological and or physical dependence, and tolerance to its effects develop quickly.

drug interactions
Ionamin can counteract the effect of drugs for high blood pressure, and some drugs used to regulate heart rhythms. It can be additive and increase the likelihood of side effects when used with decongestants or nasal sprays and drugs for asthma.

see essay
Stimulants and Drugs for Weight Loss.

Ismelin

generic name

guanethidine

action and uses
A potent drug for treatment of moderate to severe high blood pressure. It acts to block the nerves which cause the arterial blood vessels to constrict. It is usually reserved for use when less potent drugs such as Inderal or Aldomet are not effective. It is customarily used with some type of diuretic. It is long acting and its effects may continue for days to weeks after discontinuing.

adult dosage
The dose varies widely, from 5 to 100 mg daily. It is usually started at a low dose and gradually increased every 3-7 days until the desired effect is obtained.

adverse effects
Ismelin has a higher incidence of side effects than many antihypertensive drugs. It can cause a rapid fall in blood pressure, and therefore dizziness, with sudden changes in position. This is most noticeable early in the morning. Diarrhea may occur, and changes in sexual function are frequent. Other less common side effects include nausea, nasal stuffiness, depression or unusual dreams.

precautions
This drug should be avoided in pregnant, potentially pregnant or nursing women and in those with ulcers.

drug interactions
Tricyclic antidepressants (Elavil, Tofranil) counteract

the effect of this drug, as do the decongestants in some allergy and cough/cold medicines and nasal sprays. Stimulants and weight control drugs also have this effect. This drug can also increase the effect of alcohol.

see essay *Drugs for High Blood Pressure.*

Isopto Carpine

generic name

> pilocarpine

action and uses An eye drop preparation used for treatment of glaucoma. Glaucoma is an often hereditary disease of the eye in which the normal flow of fluid through the chambers of the eye is obstructed and pressure within the eye increases. The increased pressure can gradually (or suddenly in acute glaucoma) cause blindness. When applied to the eye, pilocarpine causes the pupil to constrict and this subsequently causes a fall in pressure inside the eye. This effect takes place within 15-30 minutes and lasts four to eight hours.

adult dosage Initially, one drop of a 0.25-1% solution is placed in the eye every 6-8 hours, and the concentration and dose are adjusted individually.

adverse effects Occasionally aching over the eye or decreased vision in the dark, local irritation and allergic reactions may occur. If an excessive dose is used, other effects such as sweating, slowed heart rate or gastrointestinal disturbance may occur.

precautions It is important to avoid contaminating the eye drop container by not touching the eye on application, and keeping the lid tightly closed. If more than one eye medicine is being used, they should be carefully marked.

drug interactions Since pilocarpine is a cholinergic drug, its action can be counteracted by excessive doses of the many anticholinergic-antispasmodic drugs such as Pro-Banthine, antihistamines, or tricyclic antidepressants such as Elavil.

Isordil

generic name

> isosorbide dinitrate (available by generic name)

action and uses A drug used to relieve pain in the treatment of angina pectoris, a heart condition characterized by pain (usually after exercise or emotion) in the chest or arm. The pain is

189

due to lack of oxygen carried by the blood. Isordil acts in two ways: to open up the (often partly blocked) blood vessels to the heart, and to dilate peripheral blood vessels to decrease the work the heart must do.

Isordil is also sometimes used to treat conditions where blood circulation is poor, such as Raynaud's disease, and in certain other heart failure conditions.

adult dosage
For acute attacks the usual dosage is 2.5 to 10 mg; the tablets are placed under the tongue and allowed to dissolve. The tablets each contain either 2.5 mg or 5 mg. For regular use tablets containing 5 mg, 10 mg, or 20 mg are *swallowed* to reduce the frequency of anginal attacks. For this purpose the usual dosage is 5-30 mg taken four times per day by swallowing. Long-acting tablets and long-acting capsules, containing 40 mg isosorbide dinitrate are also available. These should be taken every 6 to 12 hours.

adverse effects
Flushing is very common and is due to increased blood flow to the skin. Throbbing headache often occurs and is also associated with changes in blood flow. A feeling of faintness or dizziness can occur (particularly in hot weather) more commonly in persons with high blood pressure.

precautions
If more than 2 or 3 tablets do not relieve the pain, the doctor should be notified at once.

drug interactions
Excessive alcohol intake tends to dilate blood vessels and increase the action of nitroglycerin-like drugs, as do certain antihypertensive drugs, such as Apresoline.

see essays
Drugs Used to Prevent or Treat Circulation Problems. Drugs for Angina Pectoris.

Isosorbide dinitrate (generic name). See ISORDIL, SORBITRATE.

Isoxsuprine (generic name). See VASODILAN.

Keflex

generic name

cephalexin

action and uses
An antibiotic which is similar chemically and in its actions to penicillins. It is one of a group of drugs widely used (and now thought to be overused) in hospitals called cephalosporins. The proper primary use of Keflex is as a substitute

for ampicillin when allergy to the penicillin group of antibiotics is present or when a bacterium such as *Klebsiella* is especially sensitive to it. It is used more widely, however, in a variety of infections of the urinary tract, chest and elsewhere, although often less costly drugs are equally effective.

adult dosage   Usually 250 mg – 500 mg every six hours on an empty stomach. The maximum dose is 4 grams per day. Keflex should be taken regularly for the number of days recommended (usually 7-10 days) to be fully effective and to prevent recurrence of infection and development of resistance.

adverse effects   Some people are allergic to Keflex and may develop skin rashes, itching or difficulty in breathing. Those persons who have had severe allergies to penicillin are more likely to be allergic to Keflex. Keflex may also cause nausea, other stomach problems, or diarrhea since it also can effect the bacteria in the lower gastrointestinal tract. More rarely, it can cause headaches, dizziness, changes in the blood, and abnormalities in the kidney.

precautions   A person who has had a severe (anaphylactoid) reaction to penicillin should probably not take Keflex. Pregnant, potentially pregnant and nursing women should use caution in taking this drug.

drug interactions   The likelihood of damage to the kidneys is increased if Keflex is taken with the diuretic Lasix, as well as certain other antibiotics, such as gentamicin (Garamycin). Keflex can increase the effect of the anticoagulant Coumadin to increase the risk of bleeding.

see essay   *Drugs to Treat Infections.*

Kenalog Cream and Ointment

generic name

triamcinolone (available by generic name)

action and uses   A commonly used topical preparation of a synthetic corticosteroid, or cortisone-like drug. It is used primarily because of its anti-inflammatory effects in the treatment of many types of skin disorders such as psoriasis, certain types of neurodermatitis and a variety of other conditions, where there is no infection. In many cases, the effects are dramatic. Because it retards formation of scar tissue, it can also prevent scarring.

adult dosage   The 0.025-0.1% preparation is applied sparingly 2-3 times daily. It is available in ointment and cream in several strengths, depending upon where it is to be used.

adverse effects

If the preparation is not used for long periods or on infected areas, there are virtually no important adverse effects; however, if the preparations are used for long intervals on the face, they can cause eruptions and redness. If Kenalog preparations are used for long periods on a large portion of the body, the corticosteroid can be absorbed and get into the body. This can cause weight gain, ulcers or stomach upset, decreased resistance to infection and stress, and can be quite hazardous. If used on an infected area of the skin it can help the infection spread, and it can be very hazardous if used for any viral skin lesions such as herpes (cold sores), shingles or chickenpox.

precautions

Do not use without a physician's specific instructions, and use only on affected areas. Do not use on a skin area which appears infected without consulting a physician.

drug interactions

No significant interactions will occur although other topical preparations placed on the same skin area may interfere with effects.

see essays

Steroids or Cortisone-like Drugs. Drugs for Skin and Local Disorders.

Kwell

generic name

gamma benzene hexachloride

action and uses

A liquid medication used to treat scabies and lice. Kwell kills both scabies, which are microscopic-sized parasites that get into the skin, and lice which live and multiply in areas of the body covered by hair. It is only effective when combined with other measures to eliminate the parasites and their eggs, including careful laundering of clothes, bedding and other personal items.

adult dosage

Kwell comes as a lotion, a cream and a shampoo. It is either shampooed into the affected area, or applied for a brief period. It should not be left on the skin for long periods.

adverse effects

Kwell can produce a red eruption on the skin where it is applied due to local irritation or allergic reactions. It can produce hazardous effects on the liver and blood cells if left on large body areas for a long time, or ingested.

precautions

Kwell is a poison if taken by mouth and must be kept out

of the reach of small children. It should not be applied repeatedly or left on the skin for long periods.

drug interactions None have been reported.

see essay *Drugs for Skin and Local Disorders.*

Lanoxin (brand name for digoxin). See DIGOXIN.

Larotid

generic name

amoxicillin (available by generic name)

action and uses An antibiotic used to treat many infections including those of the urinary tract, ear, nose and throat. It is one of several so-called "semi-synthetic" penicillins which is made by both chemical and biological manipulations of penicillin produced by the mold *penicillium*.

Amoxicillin, like penicillin, acts by preventing bacteria from forming their cell walls. They therefore break up. It has no effect on human cells since they have a different structure. Though basic penicillin G is still one of the most important of all the antibiotics, it has several disadvantages. One is the somewhat limited effectiveness against the Gram negative organisms. Another disadvantage is that it is not totally effective when taken by mouth because penicillin G is broken down by stomach acid. Amoxicillin is highly effective when given by mouth because it is not broken down by stomach acid. It differs from ampicillin only in that it may be taken in the presence or absence of food, and it is more costly.

Because it is active against many kinds of bacteria, it is called a "broad spectrum" antibiotic. It is less effective than penicillin G against Gram positive cocci (found in abcesses and ear infections), but more effective against Gram negative bacteria which cause urinary tract infections. It is not effective against fungal or viral diseases. Antibiotics should not be used for trivial infections or to treat non-sensitive bacteria; such use only produces resistant bacteria which are difficult to eliminate.

adult dosage The average adult dose is 250 mg or 500 mg every 6 hours . The dosage should always be advised by a physician and will vary with the type and severity of infection.

adverse effects Many people develop allergic reactions to the penicillin group of drugs. Once sensitization develops, *all* forms of penicillin including amoxicillin can produce a reaction. An allergic reaction is characterized by either skin rashes, hives, itching, fever, difficulty in breathing, or swelling of the lips and tongue. Persons who have infectious mononucleosis often develop rashes due to ampicillin and should not take it while they are ill with the disease. Amoxicillin can also produce stomach upset due to the killing of certain bacteria in the intestine and may cause diarrhea. It may also cause mild fungus infections of the anorectal area or vagina.

precautions This antibiotic should not be used if there is a history of allergy to any type of penicillin. Due to a high frequency of rash, it should not be taken by persons with infectious mononucleosis. Once a course of amoxicillin is begun, it should be taken for its entire course of not less than 5-7 days, unless of course side effects occur. It should not be stopped when the infection seems to be gone, since the infection can recur. The frequent starting and stopping of any antibiotic only leads to the development of resistant bacteria which are much more difficult to treat. Pregnant, potentially pregnant and nursing women should use with caution.

drug interactions The effectiveness of amoxicillin may be hindered by the antibiotics erythromycin and chloramphenicol, if they are used together.

see essay *Drugs to Treat Infections.*

Lasix

generic name

furosemide

action and uses A potent diuretic ("water pill") used to treat excessive retention of water, for example, in congestive heart failure and in some forms of kidney disease. Lasix is also sometimes used for high blood pressure, but it offers no particular advantage over the less potent diuretics, such as hydrochlorothiazide, which work on a different part of the kidney. Its primary action is to promote the loss of excess salt and water via the kidneys, thus relieving edema (the swelling of body tissue due to fluid retention).

adult dosage Usually 20-80 mg per day taken as a single morning dose, or in divided doses. Higher doses are sometimes needed. The diuretic response is usually seen within one to two hours.

adverse effects

Lasix can cause excessive loss of potassium, especially when taken daily. If this occurs potassium can be replaced either in the diet (orange juice, tomato juice, bananas or dried fruit) or with liquid potassium chloride (KCl). Lasix also tends to cause an increased blood sugar in those predisposed to diabetes and may increase uric acid levels (the substance in the blood which can cause gout). If used to excess, Lasix or any diuretic can cause dehydration and may effect kidney function and the amount of waste products in the blood. Therefore, the initial use of Lasix is usually followed carefully to avoid these effects.

precautions

This drug should be used with caution by pregnant or potentially pregnant women, and by patients with gout or diabetes.

drug interactions

Taken in conjunction with cortisone-like drugs, such as prednisone, it can cause excessive potassium loss. Potentially serious interactions may also occur if Lasix is taken in conjunction with digitalis drugs for the heart (Lanoxin, digoxin), because if and when too much potassium is eliminated from the system by the Lasix, the heart can become sensitive to the toxic effects of digitalis. Medical supervision is essential.

see essays

Drugs for High Blood Pressure. Diuretics.

Librax

generic
ingredients

```
tranquilizer = chlordiazepoxide
antispasmodic = clidinium
```

Librax is a popular combination drug used in the treatment of peptic ulcer and other types of gastrointestinal spasm. Like many other similar preparations, it combines an antichoiinergic-antispasmodic compound, which decreases the contraction of the bowel and stomach, with a commonly used tranquilizer, in this case Librium. Apparently it is assumed that the bowel symptoms are associated with anxiety and thus can be relieved by a tranquilizer. Whether in fact the combination is more effective than an antispasmodic alone is not known.

adult dosage

The usual dose is 1-2 capsules 3-4 times per day, adjusted according to clinical response.

adverse effects

Both components of this preparation have side effects. The Librium can cause drowsiness, dizziness or confusion, especially in older persons. If taken for long periods and then discontinued, withdrawal symptoms of anxiety,

195

insomnia and nightmares can occur. The antispasmodic clidinium can cause dry mouth, bladder dysfunction (usually in persons with prostate problems) or blurring vision.

precautions

Lower doses may be necessary in older persons, in those sensitive to tranquilizing drugs, and in those persons with prostate trouble or glaucoma. If drowsiness occurs, driving or operating machinery may be hazardous. Librax should be avoided by pregnant and potentially pregnant women.

drug dependence

Prolonged use of Librax has the potential to cause dependence, and there may be withdrawal symptoms if discontinued suddenly.

drug interactions

The Librium in this combination can add to the effects of alcohol and tranquilizers and sedatives. The clidinium can be additive (and cause excessive dry mouth or constipation) to other antispasmodic drugs, antihistamines, some cough/cold medicines as well as some tricyclic antidepressants such as Elavil.

see essays

Drugs for Nausea, Stomach Upset and Ulcers. Minor Tranquilizers.

Librium

generic name

chlordiazepoxide (available by generic name)

action and uses

A minor tranquilizer widely used to treat anxiety and nervousness. The primary effect of Librium is to produce calm and decrease the feeling of anxiety. Librium, together with related drugs such as Valium, Serax, Dalmane and Tranxene, is one of a group of drugs which are the most frequently prescribed in the United States. Librium is usually prescribed to relieve the symptoms of a condition in the same way that narcotics are used to relieve pain. In general it has no effect on the cause of the symptoms. Librium is also often used in the treatment of withdrawal from certain drugs, especially alcohol. It can also be used as a sleeping medication in a similar way to the related drug, Dalmane. It is not known exactly how these drugs work.

adult dosage

The usual dose of Librium ranges from 10 mg per day to 10-25 mg, 3 to 4 times per day, depending on individual requirements. Some people are strongly sedated by 10-20 mg, while others are not especially affected by that dose.

adverse effects

The most common side effect of Librium is sedation (tiredness) and depression, and sometimes, dizziness, but

196

this can usually be relieved by lowering the dosage. Other side effects are relatively uncommon. A few individuals may suffer from increased anxiety when taking Librium, but this is rare. When Librium is taken in combination with alcohol the two drugs act together and marked sedation may occur. In some cases the sedation may interfere with working and driving.

precautions

There is a possibility that minor tranquilizers may cause birth defects and the manufacturers therefore warn against the use of Librium in prgnant or potentially pregnant women.

drug
dependence

Librium is not addictive in the same way as narcotics but, like other sedatives, it can be habit-forming to a certain extent if taken for a long period of time. If it is then stopped suddenly some withdrawal symptoms may occur, especially after large doses. These can include anxiety, insomnia and nightmares.

drug interactions

Librium can enhance the sedative effect of alcohol, antihistamines, sleeping pills and narcotics, sometimes to a dangerous extent. Unlike many sedatives, Librium does not interfere with the actions of the anticoagulant Coumadin.

see essay

Minor Tranquilizers.

Lidex

generic name

fluocinonide (available by generic name)

action and uses

A commonly used topical preparation of a synthetic corticosteroid, or cortisone-like drug. It is used primarily because of its anti-inflammatory effects in the treatment of many types of skin disorders such as psoriasis, certain types of neurodermatitis and a variety of other conditions which are not infected. In many cases, the effects are dramatic. Because it retards formation of scar tissue, it can also prevent scarring.

adult dosage

The 0.05% preparation is applied sparingly 3-4 times daily. It is available in both ointment and cream in several strengths, depending upon where it is used.

adverse effects

If the preparation is not used for long periods or on infected areas, there are virtually no important adverse effects; however, if the preparations are used for long intervals on the face, they can cause eruptions and redness. If Lidex preparations are used for long periods on a large portion of the body, the corticosteroid can be absorbed and get into the body. This can cause weight gain, ulcers or stomach upset, decreased resistance to infection and stress, and can be quite hazardous. If used on an infected area of the skin it can help the infection spread, and it can be very hazardous if used for any viral skin lesions such as herpes (cold sores), shingles or chickenpox.

precautions

Do not use without a physician's specific instructions, and use only on affected areas. Do not use on a skin area which appears infected without consulting a physician.

drug interactions

No significant interactions will occur although other topical preparations placed on the same skin area may interfere with effects.

see essays

Steroids or Cortisone-like Drugs. Drugs for Skin and Local Disorders.

Lomotil

generic ingredients

> antidiarrheal = diphenoxylate
> antispasmodic = atropine

action and uses

A drug used to treat diarrhea. Since its introduction in 1961, it has become increasingly popular with overseas travelers as a medication for this very common hazard of traveling. One of its two components, diphenoxylate, is a synthetic narcotic similar to Demerol. At normal doses of Lomotil, this ingredient does not produce the euphoria, pain relief or dependence associated with Demerol. It does, however, act like morphine to decrease the movement of the bowel, and thus decrease diarrhea. The other ingredient, atropine, is added because it too has a constipating effect, and because its presence is supposed to discourage any possible drug abuse with Lomotil. However, the actual amount of atropine in Lomotil is probably too small to have any significant effect except when the medication is taken in overdose. Interestingly enough, many authorities have expressed the opinion that, although Lomotil can be effective on a short-term basis, continued use when traveller's diarrhea occurs can prolong certain diarrheal illnesses by allowing retention of the toxins or bacteria in the bowel.

adult dosage

Initially, one or two 2.5 mg tablets, followed by a single 2.5 mg tablet every 4-6 hours until diarrhea stops.

adverse effects

Lomotil can cause dry mouth, nausea and dizziness. In

excessive amounts, it can cause vomiting, sedation, depression, along with signs of atropine poisoning (flushed skin, fever). Allergic reactions may rarely occur.

precautions

Lomotil should be used with caution by patients with glaucoma or prostate trouble. If diarrhea persists for more than a few days, the cause should be investigated.

drug dependence

Because of the presence of diphenoxylate, Lomotil may be capable of causing psychological and or physical dependence, but only when taken daily over an extended period.

drug interactions

Oversedation may rarely result from concurrent use of Lomotil and sedatives, sleeping pills, tranquilizers or alcohol. Certain antihistamines and antidepressants can be additive to the antispasmodic affects of Lomotil.

see essay

Drugs for Diarrhea.

Lo Ovral

generic ingredients

progestogen = norgestrel
estrogen = ethinyl estradiol

action and uses

Lo Ovral is one of many combination birth control pills made up of an estrogen compound and a progesterone-like compound. This newer pill, which contains 60% of the hormones in Ovral, differs from many other birth control pills in that it contains a lower dose of estrogen, which tends to alter its effects somewhat. Recent studies have suggested that lower doses of estrogen in birth control pills such as Lo Ovral may be associated with fewer side effects. However, the lower dose of estrogen also results in a greater incidence of "breakthrough" or mid-cycle bleeding, which in turn may be a cause for greater dropout rate and therefore lesser effectiveness as a contraceptive. This effect often decreases with more prolonged use. At present, its effectiveness in contraception appears to be similar to the higher-dose birth control pills.

adult dosage

In general, one tablet is taken daily (usually at night) on the first cycle beginning on the 5th day of menstruation and continuing for 21 days. The pill is then discontinued for 7 days and restarted on the eigth day for another 21-day cycle.

adverse effects

Use of oral contraceptive pills has been associated with a variety of side effects. Lo Ovral may be associated with a higher incidence of breakthrough bleeding or spotting, but it appears to produce a slightly decreased incidence (as

199

compared with some other higher estrogen-containing pills) of effects of estrogen excess, such as nausea, edema and leg cramps. Other minor side effects include acne, breast discomfort, depression, gastrointestinal upset, headaches and vaginal infections. More significant but less common side effects include the risk of thrombophlebitis, increased blood pressure, increased blood sugar and gallbladder disease. The risk of certain side effects such as heart disease and gallbladder disease appear to increase with age (especially over the age of 35) while a history of true migraine headaches is associated with increased headaches and risk (though small) of stroke. A history of heavy smoking is associated with increased risk of heart disease, particularly in the age group over 40.

precautions
A history of thrombophlebitis, blood clots, and migraine headaches is usually a relative contraindication to the use of oral contraceptives. For women with other risk factors, such as age over 35, a history of heavy smoking, gallbladder disease, diabetes or high blood pressure, use should be weighed carefully against alternative birth control methods.

drug interactions
Several drug interactions have been suggested but none have been well-documented as significant in most cases.

see essays
Hormonal Drugs. Oral Contraceptives.

Macrodantin

generic name

nitrofurantoin (available by generic name)

action and uses
An antibacterial drug used to treat infections of the kidneys, bladder and urinary system. Macrodantin is specifically designed to treat urinary infections and is not customarily used against any other infections. It is active against many of the bacterial infections which commonly affect the urinary tract, but there are a few bacteria which are resistant to Macrodantin. It is the same chemical as Furadantin but is made in larger crystals and is therefore absorbed more slowly into the system. This form was developed to decrease the gastrointestinal distress often associated with Furadantin.

adult dosage
Usually 50-100 mg, four times a day. Macrodantin can be given with food or milk. It should be taken for the full period of time directed, unless adverse effects occur.

adverse effects
The most common side effects are nausea, vomiting and

diarrhea. These are reduced if the drug is taken with milk or other food. Some people may develop allergies to Macrodantin and may suffer from rashes, hives, fever, chills, cough or other symptoms. This drug can cause serious effects on nerve function, especially in those with diabetes, kidney disease, or serious chronic disease. It can also cause lung scarring and effects on red blood cells.

precautions
Macrodantin should not be used in pregnancy, in patients with kidney diseases, severe diabetics, or persons with G6PD deficiency (a red blood cell disease). Because of the potential for serious reactions, its use should be carefully supervised.

drug interactions
Macrodantin blocks the effect of nalidixic acid (Neg-Gram), which is also used to treat urinary infections, and therefore the two drugs should not be taken together.

see essay
Drugs to Treat Infections.

Marax

generic
ingredients

bronchodilators = theophylline
ephedrine
antihistamine/sedative = hydroxyzine

action and uses
A combination of two drugs which relax the bronchi, plus hydroxyzine used to treat asthma. Theophylline and ephedrine both act on the muscles of the bronchi, relax them, and open up the airways. Hydroxyzine theoretically provides a mild sedative for anxious asthmatic patients and counteracts any stimulant effect of the ephedrine. However, neither effect is proven or even likely at the small dose of hydroxyzine used. It is contended by some that the hydroxyzine has a beneficial antihistamine effect, but this is unproven. Most often, theophylline alone in proper doses is equally effective, less costly, and has fewer side effects. Further, this fixed combination does not allow dose adjustment.

adult dosage
1 or 2 tablets every four to six hours (to treat attacks or to prevent them).

adverse effects
Adverse effects from the ephedrine component can include nervousness, high blood pressure, fast heart rate, or paliptations. The theophylline can cause nausea, headaches or muscle cramps, and also palpitations.

precautions
This drug should be avoided by pregnant and potentially pregnant women. Marax should be used cautiously in people who have heart disease or high blood pressure. It

can be additive to certain over-the-counter drugs for asthma so the prescribing physician should be aware of all drugs being used, including aerosols or inhalers.

drug
interactions

The ephedrine can be additive (and thus increase side effects) to drugs for coughs and colds, but can counteract antihypertensive drugs. The theophylline can interact with anticoagulant drugs like Coumadin.

see essay

Drugs for Asthma and Lung Disease.

Meclizine (generic name). See ANTIVERT.

Medrol

generic name

methylprednisolone

action and uses

Medrol is one of several drugs referred to as "steroids" or "corticosteroids." Corticosteroids are hormones produced by the cortex of the adrenal glands. Drugs with very similar properties to these hormones can also be made by chemical synthesis. Medrol is one of these "synthetic" steroid hormones, used in a wide variety of disorders usually associated with severe inflammation and/or destruction of tissue, such as acute arthritis or serious allergic reactions, as in severe asthma. Medrol is very similar to prednisone, although it is much more costly, but it may have slightly fewer side effects.

Medrol and related corticosteroids act on many cells in the body to change the production of proteins and the way cells handle carbohydrates and fats, and certain minerals. This produces several desirable effects when the drug is given in higher doses. First, it acts to suppress inflammation, which can be useful in certain types of arthritis (although it is used as a last resort in this situation); in inflammatory disease of the bowel, such as ulcerative colitis; and in a large variety of skin diseases where there is inflammation of the skin, such as psoriasis, or eczema. Secondly, it acts to suppress certain types of white blood cells and lowers the body's immunity, which can be useful in the treatment of certain types of "auto-immune" diseases (where the body reacts to its own tissues) such as lupus erythematosus, certain types of leukemia where there is an overproduction of the white blood cells as well as in the prevention of rejection of transplanted organs. Thirdly, it acts to inhibit allergic reactions in severe allergic conditions such as asthma, and serious skin allergies such as poison ivy and poison oak. Medrol has a variety of other actions which are sometimes used in treatment, but more often cause adverse effects as noted below.

adult dosage The dose is highly individualized and may be as high as 100 mg or more a day, or as little as 5 mg per day. When first started, it is often taken in high doses, sometimes several times a day, but when taken chronically, it is usually taken once daily in the morning, or once every other day, depending on the circumstances.

adverse effects The adverse effects of Medrol are related to both the dose and the length of time the drug is taken. A single dose of any amount may usually be taken without significant adverse effects. However, the incidence of serious adverse effects increases considerably with time at any dose greater than the physiological equivalent (approximately 7.5 mg per day). The most common adverse reaction observed in a large series of hospitalized patients on the similar drug prednisone included disturbances of water and salt to produce edema (or water retention) and loss of potassium (which can cause weakness), but because it has less effect on salt and water, Medrol is believed to cause fewer problems of this type.

Other common side effects include development of abnormal fat deposits around the face ("moon face"), neck ("buffalo chump") or abdomen, weight gain, increased bruising, gastrointestinal bleeding and/or upset, mental confusion, and diabetes. Antacids are frequently given to prevent the gastrointestinal problems. A continuing effect is the decreased susceptibility to infections and often the masking of the symptoms of these infections. For this reason, those with a history of, or exposure to chronic infections such as tuberculosis are observed carefully. With longer use, there is often gradual degeneration of bone and muscle which can cause fractures and muscle weakness, and cataracts may develop. Obviously, the use of this drug for long periods requires very careful analysis of benefits versus risks. It has been found that certain, but not all, chronic ailments which require this drug for very long periods can be controlled by giving Medrol every other day. This is desirable whenever possible since it tends to eliminate most of the severe side effects.

Another practical effect of using Medrol relates to the fact that it tends to suppress the normal effect of the adrenal gland. In stress, the adrenal gland puts out much more corticosteroid to help the body handle the stress. The absence of this extra reserve can be life threatening. A person on corticosteroids does not have this reserve, so that if an accident occurs, or surgery is required, higher doses may be needed for a few days.

precautions

Use of Medrol especially for more than seven days requires the careful supervision of a physician who should be notified of any changes which occur, especially after altering the dose, or adding any other drug. Persons taking this drug for long periods should carry a card or wear a bracelet giving this information, in the event of an emergency.

drug interactions

Medrol can interact additively with many diuretics such as hydrochlorothiazide or Lasix, to cause excessive loss of potassium, which can cause weakness. Since diuretics are often used to treat the edema caused by corticosteroids, this interaction can be anticipated and prevented by supplementing the potassium intake. Since aspirin and several other anti-inflammatory drugs, such as Motrin, used to treat arthritis, also cause gastric upset and ulcer, they may be additive to this effect of prednisone.

see essay

Steroids or Cortisone-like Drugs.

Medroxyprogesterone (generic name). See PROVERA.

Mellaril

generic name

thioridazine

action and uses

A major tranquilizer used to treat disorders of thinking and anxiety. Mellaril is one of a group of tranquilizers, including Thorazine and Stelazine, which have been widely used to treat conditions in which a person's perception of reality is disturbed. This disturbance may cause a person to think he is in a different time or place (disorientation), or that he can fly (a delusion), or that he hears voices or sees visions (hallucinations). Mellaril is used to treat these disturbances in conditions such as schizophrenia, manic-depression, severe alcohol withdrawal and some neurological disorders such as multiple sclerosis. It is also used to treat patients who have taken LSD and amphetamines. Mellaril has the effect of "returning to reality" a person with disordered thinking, but it has little effect on normal thinking. Mellaril also has sedative effects, but is not used primarily for this. It is sometimes preferred over similar drugs because it causes fewer neurological side effects.

adult dosage

For the treatment of thought disorders, the initial dose of Mellaril may be 25-200 mg per day, eventually rising to 800 mg per day in some cases. The dose is likely to be highly individualized, because sensitivity to the drug varies widely from person to person. Generally speaking, however, the dose tends to be lower for older people, and, whatever the a patient's age, it may usually be taken just once a day (often at bedtime, to take advantage of its sedative effect) when used over a long period of time.

adverse effects

Mellaril may produce a number of significant side effects, and can occasionally cause serious drug reactions. Its use, therefore, must be carefully supervised. When first taken, it is likely to produce heavy sedation, a sensation of mental dullness, and, in some cases, blurred vision, dry mouth and constipation. These effects usually diminish if the drug is continued for two to three weeks or more. Mellaril also lowers the blood pressure, an effect which may manifest itself in a sensation of dizziness when a person stands up suddenly. In some people, Mellaril can cause restlessness, a fixed facial expression, and trembling in the hands, arms or legs. These side effects, which ressemble the symptoms of Parkinson's disease, can usually be controlled with an anti-Parkinsonian drug like Cogentin. A few people who have taken Mellaril for a long time experience an involuntary movement of the tongue and lips. Occasionally, Mellaril can cause a skin rash, jaundice, or a decrease in the white blood cell count which increases the patient's vulnerability to infection and the drug must be discontinued.

precautions

Prolonged use requires regular medical evaluation at intervals. There may be some interference with driving or operating machinery.

drug interactions

Oversedation is possible when Mellaril is taken in combination with alcohol, other sedatives and tranquilizers, sleeping pills, antidepressants, antihistamines and drugs containing narcotics. If taken with the antihypertensive drugs Ismelin and Aldomet it can counteract their blood pressure-lowering effect. It can also cause constipation or bladder dysfunction in some if combined with antispasmodic drugs, anti-Parkinson drugs like Cogentin and tricyclic antidepressants like Elavil.

see essay

Major Tranquilizers.

Meprobamate

trade names

Equanil, Miltown

action and uses A minor tranquilizer used to relieve mild tension and anxiety. Both Equanil and Miltown (other trade names for meprobamate) are very similar to barbiturates in their sedative effects. Their use as sedatives however, has diminished somewhat since the introduction of Librium and Valium. Meprobamate is also frequently used in cases of muscle strain (as in back strain) as a muscle relaxant. Whether its beneficial effect in such cases is due to sedation or to true muscle relaxation is not clear.

adult dosage Usually 200-400 mg four times a day and sometimes double that dose.

adverse effects The incidence of allergic reactions to meprobamate is significant. Such reactions may include skin rashes or hives. Other common side effects may include nausea, headache, dizziness and excessive drowsiness.

precautions Meprobamate should not be taken by pregnant, potentially pregnant or nursing women. It may interfere with driving or operating machinery.

drug dependence Meprobamate can produce psychological and or physical dependence. Once habituation to the drug has developed, convulsions can occur if the drug is suddenly stopped, especially if the daily dose has been more than 800 mg four times a day.

drug interactions Meprobamate sedative effects can be increased by alcohol, other sedatives and tranquilizers, sleeping pills and antidepressants. It can decrease the effects of anticoagulants, oral contraceptives, and the estrogens used in hormone replacement therapy, because it affects the way the liver metabolizes these drugs.

see essay *Minor Tranquilizers.*

Minocin

generic name

minocycline

action and uses A newer and slightly different member of one of the most commonly used oral antibiotic groups, the tetracyclines. There are a number of tetracycline drugs available, but most are comparable in their actions and side effects except for Minocin and Vibramycin. In general, the tetracyclines are known as "broad spectrum" antibiotics because they can be used in a wide variety of different infections, although they are first choice drugs in very few common infections. They act by stopping the production of proteins in sensitive bacterial cells with little effect on human cells. Minocin is currently very commonly used in low doses to inhibit the bacteria on the face which are believed to contribute to acne. It is also frequently used by those with chronic bronchitis or other lung disease. It has no effect on viral illnesses, including colds, or fungus infections. Minocycline is distinguished from other tetracyclines by its longer action, requiring less frequent dosing, its somewhat greater safety in persons with kidney disease, and a higher incidence of vertigo as well as a higher cost.

adult dosage

The dosing of Minocin is different from other tetracyclines. The usual adult dose is 200 mg initially, then 100 mg every 12 hours for a prescribed number of days as specified by the physician. It is very important to take this on an empty stomach. The dose may vary in some cases such as acne, where it may be lower.

adverse effects

Minocycline can cause various gastrointestinal symptoms including nausea and vomiting, burning stomach or belching, cramps and diarrhea. The latter symptom is often due to the fact that tetracyclines inhibit some bacteria in the lower intestine and elsewhere and allow overgrowth of other bacteria and minor fungi. These symptoms may be less frequent with Minocycline.

Normally the symptoms tend to disappear when the drug is discontinued. Less commonly, minocycline can cause rashes, or other allergic reactions and sensitivity of the skin to sunlight causing rashes (photosensitivity). It can also tend to worsen certain types of kidney disease, and rarely cause liver damage or blood cell abnormalities.

precautions

Minocycline should not be taken by pregnant or potentially pregnant or nursing women, and should be used with caution when significant liver disease is present. This antibiotic, like all others, should be taken for the time period directed, and every dose should be taken. Failure to do this can result in inadequate treatment of the infection, recurrence or development of resistant infections.

drug interactions

The most common interaction is between the tetracyclines and antacids or milk products, since the tetracycline binds to these in the stomach and does not get into the body. Minocycline can potentially increase the effect of the anticoagulant Coumadin and increase the hazard of bleeding.

see essay   *Drugs to Treat Infections.*

Monistat

generic name

> miconazole

action and uses   An antifungal cream used to treat fungus or yeast infections of the vagina. Monistat is effective in killing several fungi, including the one called *Candida* which most commonly infects the vagina. This kind of infection causes a thin, itchy discharge, and often occurs after broad spectrum antibiotic therapy, or in diabetes.

adult dosage   The cream is usually applied at bedtime for 10-14 days with a measured dose applicator. It is important to use the drug for the full period of time, since otherwise recurrent infections will occur.

adverse effects   The most common side effects relate to occasional local irritation or burning. Sometimes allergic reactions may occur.

precautions   It is currently believed that Monistat is safe in the last six months of pregnancy but earlier use should be avoided.

drug interactions   None are currently known.

see essay   *Drugs for Skin and Local Disorders.*

Motrin

generic name

> ibuprofen

action and uses   One of several recently introduced drugs used to treat various types of arthritis. It has some ability to relieve pain and also acts to decrease inflammation. Motrin, like the other recently introduced drugs with similar actions such as Tolectin, Naprosyn and Nalfon, is often used as an alternative to aspirin in the therapy of osteoarthritis, rheumatoid and other types of arthritis. In some cases, its effect is seen in a few days; and in other cases such as chronic osteoarthritis, its effects may be seen only after a period of use. Because of its considerably greater cost, it is usually reserved for those persons on whom aspirin is not effective or is not tolerated.

adult dosage   The currently recommended dose is 300-400 mg three to four times daily usually adjusted according to response.

adverse effects

The most commonly occurring side effects are gastrointestinal irritation, occurring in 4-16% of patients, some of whom experience bleeding. Other side effects include dizziness, headaches, rash, decreased appetite and fluid retention. It can also cause visual changes.

precautions

Motrin should be avoided by pregnant, potentially pregnant and nursing women. Motrin should be used with caution in those persons with heart failure and history of peptic ulcer. If bleeding or visual changes occur, the physician prescribing should be notified at once.

drug interactions

Motrin may possibly interact with anticoagulant drugs such as Coumadin and predispose to bleeding. The use of aspirin with Motrin may decrease the effectiveness of Motrin, and their stomach irritant effects can be additive.

see essay

Drugs for Pain with Inflammation.

Mycolog

generic
ingredients

antibiotics = nystatin,
neomycin sulfate,
gramicidin
steroid = triamcinolone acetonide

action and uses

A combination product used to treat local infections of the skin, Mycolog combines three antibiotics and a steroid or cortisone-like drug. Each of the antibiotics acts against different types of bacteria, or fungi. The steroid acts to reduce inflammation and irritation. The ointment is used in a variety of skin irritations with mild infection. This type of mixture has been criticized because it represents "shotgun" therapy when one specific ingredient may often be adequate.

adult dosage

Available as a cream, ointment, lotion and suspension, which are usually applied two to four times per day.

adverse effects

Allergy to any of the ingredients of Mycolog may occur and skin conditions may worsen rather than improve. This is particularly true of neomycin which has a high rate of allergic reactions. The steroid may rarely worsen infections, especially if caused by a virus, as in shingles. Serious adverse effects can occur from all the ingredients if the preparation is used on large areas for a long time, due to absorption. Also, resistant bacteria or fungi can appear and cause reinfection.

precautions

The topical Mycolog should not be used over large parts of the body at any one time. It should not be used to treat the sores of "cold sore" or on smallpox vaccinations or chickenpox sores.

drug interactions   If used properly, drug interactions are not a problem.

see essays   *Drugs to Treat Infections. Drugs for Skin and Local Disorders. Steroids or Cortisone-like Drugs.*

Mycostatin

generic name

> nystatin (available by generic name)

action and uses   An antibiotic used to treat fungus infections. Mycostatin is not active against infections caused by bacteria, but is effective in treating many fungus infections, particularly those caused by a family of fungi known as *Candida*. This causes moniliasis, an infection which can affect the vagina to produce a clear discharge, itching or burning. The mouth and anorectal area can also be affected. This often occurs after treatment with broad spectrum antibiotics or with diabetes.

adult dosage   Usually one or two tablets inserted in the vagina daily for two weeks. The tablets are supplied with an applicator and should be used regardless of intervening menstrual period. Creams, ointments, and suspensions are usable for other infections. It is very important to use them nightly for the full time period since infections may otherwise recur.

adverse effects   There are no serious side effects except for occasional minor irritations.

precautions   No special precautions are necessary with Mycostatin and it can be used during pregnancy.

drug interactions   None are known.

see essays   *Drugs to Treat Infections. Drugs for Skin and Local Disorders.*

Mystatin (generic name). See MYCOSTATIN.

Mysteclin-F

generic ingredients

> antibiotic = tetracycline
> antifungal agent = amphotericin B

action and uses   A combination of one of the most commonly used oral antibiotics, with an antifungal drug. In the generic form tetracycline was the 4th most frequently prescribed drug in

1976. There are a number of tetracycline drugs available, but most are comparable in their actions and side effects except for Minocin and Vibramycin. Tetracycline is known as a "broad spectrum" antibiotic because it can be used in a wide variety of different infections, although it is the first choice drug in very few common infections. It acts by stopping the production of proteins in sensitive bacterial cells with little effect on human cells. Tetracycline is currently very commonly used in low doses to inhibit the bacteria on the face which are believed to contribute to acne. It is also frequently used by those with chronic bronchitis or other lung disease. Less frequently it is used to treat urinary tract infections or venereal disease when penicillin allergy is present. It has no effect on viral illnesses, including colds, or fungal infections. The anti-fungal drug, amphotericin B is presumably added to prevent the growth of fungi in the intestine which can contribute to the side effects. The usefulness is not known. The amphotericin B has no effect on infections in the body since it is not absorbed from the intestine. Whether this addition is worth the extra cost is questionable.

adult dosage The usual oral dose is 250 or 500 mg every six hours for a prescribed number of days as specified by the physician. It is very important to take this on an empty stomach. The dose may vary in some cases such as acne, where it may be lower.

adverse effects Tetracycline commonly can cause various gastrointestinal symptoms including nausea and vomiting, burning stomach or belching, cramps and diarrhea. The latter symptom is often due to the fact that tetracycline also inhibits some bacteria in the lower intestine and elsewhere and allows overgrowth of other bacteria (normally held in check) and minor fungi. This can also result in vaginal infections, anorectal itching and a sore mouth (thrush). The added antifungal drug may or may not prevent this. These symptoms tend to disappear when the drug is discontinued. Less commonly, tetracycline can cause rashes, or other allergic reactions and sensitivity of the skin to sunlight causing rashes (photosensitivity). It can also tend to worsen certain types of kidney disease, and rarely cause liver damage or blood cell abnormalities. The amphotericin B has few side effects when given orally.

precautions Tetracycline should not be taken by pregnant or potentially pregnant or nursing women, and should be used with caution when significant liver or kidney disease is present.

This antibiotic, like all others, should be taken for the time period directed, and every dose should be taken. Failure to do this can result in inadequate treatment of the infection, recurrence or development of resistant infections.

drug interactions

The most common drug interaction is between tetracycline and antacids or milk products, since the tetracycline binds to these and does not get into the body. Tetracycline can potentially increase the effect of the anticoagulant Coumadin and increase the hazard of bleeding.

see essay

Drugs to Treat Infections.

Naldecon

generic ingredients

decongestants = phenylpropanolamine,
                phenylephrine
antihistamines = chlorpheniramine,
                 phenyltoloxamine

action and uses

Naldecon is a combination of two decongestant drugs related to epinephrine (phenylpropanolamine and phenylephrine) and two antihistamine drugs (chlorpheniramine and phenyltoloxamine). It is used to treat nasal congestion associated with allergy, sinusitis and the common cold. The two decongestants cut down blood flow to inflamed nasal areas and help to dry up a runny nose. The antihistamines act to prevent the action of histamine, a substance released by cells damaged by allergy or infection, which is responsible for causing the redness and inflammation experienced in allergy.

adult dosage

Naldecon is supplied as sustained action tablets and syrup. One dose (5 ml) of syrup should be taken every 4 hours; not more than 4 doses should be taken in any 24 hour period.

The sustained action tablets are formulated to be taken three times daily, at 8-hourly intervals.

adverse effects

Prolonged use may lead to a chronic runny nose condition and can be followed by a rebound congestion when Naldecon is discontinued. Because it contains two compounds related to epinephrine, Naldecon can cause palpitations and raise the blood pressure. The antihistamines in Naldecon can cause drowsiness, occasional blurring of vision, and difficulty in passing urine.

precautions

This drug should be avoided by pregnant and potentially pregnant women and nursing mothers. Naldecon may interfere with driving or using machinery. People with heart disease or high blood pressure should use this drug only after checking with their physician.

drug interactions The antihistamines can add to the sedative effects of alcohol, tranquilizers and sleeping pills. They can also add to the antispasmodic effects of drugs for gastric distress, such as Pro-Banthine and Librax, causing mouth dryness and difficulty in urinating.

The decongestants can counteract the effects of drugs for high blood pressure and cause a dangerous interaction with the MAO inhibitor drugs such as Nardil, Parnate, Eutonyl, and Eutron.

see essay *Drugs for Coughs and Colds.*

Nembutal

generic name

pentobarbital (available by generic name)

action and uses A barbiturate similar to Seconal and Butisol. Nembutal is chiefly used as a sleeping pill, although it is occasionally used as a daytime sedative to relieve anxiety and tension. It takes effect 15-30 minutes after being taken and this effect lasts 5-6 hours. When used as a sleeping medication Nembutal decreases the time it takes to go to sleep but it suppresses dreaming. After a few days tolerance can develop and it is necessary to increase the dosage to produce the same sleep inducing effect. Some of the effects of Nembutal may last longer than 5-6 hours, such as a "hangover" which may occur the morning after taking the drug.

adult dosage For sleep the usual dose is 100 mg at bedtime. If used in the daytime for relief of anxiety and tension, the usual dose is 30 mg, 2 to 4 times per day.

adverse effects When used as a sleeping pill Nembutal may cause a "hangover" effect the following morning. It may also cause a feeling of depression and tiredness, together with nausea, vomiting, and diarrhea. In older persons it may cause excitement, rather than sedation. If it is withdrawn after several weeks of use withdrawal symptoms may appear. There is often a tendency for increased dreaming and even nightmares. There may be insomnia (difficulty in sleeping) and nervousness. If the dose has been high (over 400 mg per day) seizures may occur. All these effects are due to the withdrawal of the drug. Other mild side effects of the drug include allergic skin reactions, upset stomach and muscular aches. Nembutal can suppress breathing in persons with severe lung disease.

precautions

Nembutal and other barbiturates have long been a major cause of suicidal and accidental drug overdose and death. If taken in high doses they can be very dangerous and lethal. It can be particularly dangerous if taken with alcohol or other tranquilizers.

drug dependence

If used for longer than 7 to 10 days, "tolerance" to Nembutal may develop. If this occurs dependence on the drug may develop and it it is suddenly discontinued withdrawal symptoms may occur. Therefore, it must be stopped slowly if it has been used for a long time. Because of this problem, as well as its known abuse, the prescribing of Nembutal is restricted.

drug interactions

Nembutal can interact with many other drugs, particularly the anticoagulant Coumadin to decrease its effect. Its effect is additive to the effects of other tranquilizers, sleeping pills and alcohol. The combination with any of these drugs can be very hazardous, causing suppression of breathing and even death.

see essays

Sleeping Pills. Minor Tranquilizers.

Neosporin Ophthalmic

generic ingredients

> antibiotics = neomycin,
>   polymyxin B,
>   bacitracin

action and uses

A sterile preparation for use in the eye. Neosporin is a combination of three antibiotics which between them kill a large range of bacteria. It is used short term in the treatment of infected eye conditions including conjunctivitis.

adult dosage

Supplied as ointment and drops. The ointment should be applied every 3 or 4 hours. If the drops are used, 1 or 2 drops should be instilled into the affected eye 2 to 4 times daily; it is often necessary to commence therapy by using the drops every 30 minutes.

adverse effects

As with all antibiotics, "overgrowth" of bacteria which are not sensitive to Neosporin can occur with prolonged use. Allergic reactions are not uncommon, and can be confused with the disorder being treated.

precautions

If the condition shows no improvement after a few days, or worsens, the treatment should be re-evaluated, by the physician.

see essays   *Drugs to Treat Infection. Drugs for Skin and Local Disorders.*

Nicotinic Acid (Niacin)

trade names

Nicobid, Nico-400, Nicotinex

action and uses   A vitamin of the B group which is used to lower cholesterol levels in the blood. Its effectiveness in preventing diseases associated with high blood cholesterol, such as coronary heart disease, is limited by side effects. The cholesterol lowering action is due to an effect on metabolism and transport of particles containing cholesterol (this is not related to the action of niacin in treating pellagra). In high doses, it is used to dilate blood vessels in circulation disorders, but it does not usually act on the diseased vessels, only the tiny ones such as those in the face. It is also used to treat the symptoms of pellagra (a skin condition due to niacin deficiency and characterized by light sensitivity, red blotches, diarrhea and swollen tongue). Niacin is essential for normal body function, but deficiency seldom arises as it is a normal dietary constituent, found mainly in proteins. It does not come from nicotine and does not have any effects associated with tobacco.

adult dosage   The dose recommended for the treatment of pellagra is up to 500 mg daily in divided doses.

Much higher doses are used if the drug is to be employed for lowering cholesterol levels in the blood: 2-6 grams daily, taken regularly over a long period of time.

adverse effects   In the doses given for pellagra and, particularly, for high cholesterol levels, niacin frequently produces an intense flushing of the skin, often accompanied by itching. Although this reaction decreases in intensity after several weeks' therapy, it is very unpleasant. Vomiting and diarrhea and indigestion may also occur with niacin, as well as ulcers, diabetes, liver damage and allergic reactions.

precautions   Niacin may affect uric acid and glucose levels in the blood: it should therefore be taken cautiously by persons suffering from gout, having a predisposition to diabetes, or with ulcer disease.

drug interactions   There are no significant interactions in normal doses.

see essays   *Drugs for Preventing or Treating Arteriosclerosis. Vitamins and Minerals.*

Nitrofurantoin (generic name). See MACRODANTIN.

Nitro-Bid (trade name). See NITROGLYCERIN

Nitroglycerin

trade names

> Nitro-Bid, Nitrobon, Nitroglyn, Nitrol, Nitrong, Nitrospan, Nitrostat

action and uses

A drug which is used to relieve pain in the treatment of angina pectoris, a heart condition characterized by pain (usually after exercise or emotion) in the chest or arm. The pain is due to lack of oxygen, carried by the blood. Nitroglycerin acts in two ways: to open up the (often partly blocked) blood vessels to the heart, and to dilate peripheral blood vessels to decrease the work the heart must do.

Nitroglycerin is sometimes also used to treat conditions where blood circulation is poor, such as Raynaud's disease, and in certain other heart failure conditions.

adult dosage

The tablets of nitroglycerin should be placed under the tongue and allowed to dissolve. The drug is quickly absorbed from the lining of the mouth. Up to three 0.2 mg tablets may be taken when an attack of angina pectoris occurs. The tablets may be chewed and retained in the mouth, but they should never be swallowed (if they are, absorption will be too slow to have any effect). Nitroglycerin is also available as a paste, applied in measured amounts to a skin area, usually the back. This has a more prolonged action.

adverse effects

Flushing is very common and is due to increased blood flow to the skin. Throbbing headache often occurs and is also associated with changes in blood flow. A feeling of faintness or dizziness can occur (particularly in hot weather) more commonly in persons with high blood pressure.

precautions

If more than 2 or 3 tablets do not relieve the pain, the doctor should be notified at once. Nitroglycerin tends to deteriorate in 2-6 months, so that fresh tablets should always be used. (Old tablets are not dangerous, just ineffective).

drug interactions

Excessive alcohol intake tends to dilate blood vessels and add to the action of nitroglycerin, as do certain antihypertensive drugs, such as Apresoline.

see essay

Drugs Used to Prevent or Treat Circulation Problems. Drugs for Angina Pectoris.

Norgesic

generic
ingredients

antihistamine = orphenadrine citrate pain relievers = aspirin,   phenacetin mild stimulant = caffeine

action and uses
An analgesic drug used for the relief of muscular pain. Orphenadrine is an antihistamine drug which acts in the brain to reduce muscle rigidity (it is also used to treat Parkinsonism). Aspirin and phenacetin are pain relievers which reduce the production of substances in the body responsible for causing the sensation of pain. The function of the caffeine present is not clear.

adult dosage
One or two tablets are taken 3 or 4 times daily.

adverse effects
Aspirin may cause stomach upset and irritation, and also affects the blood clotting system. Phenacetin can cause kidney damage, particularly if taken over a long period of time. Orphenadrine shares some of the side effects seen with all antihistamine drugs, including dry mouth, blurring of vision and drowsiness.

precautions
Norgesic should not be taken if you have any form of kidney disease. Because of the effects of orphenadrine, Norgesic should be used carefully if asthma, glaucoma or prostate trouble is present. Any sedative effect will be additive with alcohol or sedative drugs, including sleeping tablets and some antidepressants. When taking Norgesic, driving or operating heavy machinery may be hazardous. Norgesic should not be taken by pregnant or potentially pregnant women or nursing mothers.

drug interactions
When taken together with propoxyphene (Darvon preparations), Norgesic has been shown to cause confusion and tremors. Norgesic can add to the sedative effects of antispasmodics and antihistamines and tricyclic antidepressants.

see essay
Non-Narcotic Pain Relievers.

Norinyl 1/50

generic
ingredients

progestogen = norethindrone estrogen = mestranol

action and uses
Norinyl 1/50, which is essentially identical to Ortho-Novum 1/50, is a combination of a progesterone-like hormone and an estrogen and contains the same dose (50

micrograms) of estrogen. Recent studies have suggested that lowering the dose of estrogen may be associated with a lower incidence of estrogen-related side effects, although the incidence of breakthrough bleeding and spotting tends to be increased, especially in earlier cycles. It acts like most birth control pills to prevent contraception by affecting pituitary control of reproduction, as well as acting locally on the lining of the uterus and the cervical mucus, and possibly in other ways. When taken regularly, it is a very effective contraceptive drug.

adult dosage

In general one tablet is taken daily (usually at night) on the first cycle beginning on the 5th day of menstruation and continuing for 21 days. The pills are then discontinued for 7 days and restarted on the 8th day for another 21-day cycle.

adverse effects

Use of oral contraceptive pills has been associated with a variety of side effects. Norinyl 1/50 may be associated with a higher incidence of breakthrough bleeding or spotting, but there appears to be a slightly decreased incidence (as compared with some other higher estrogen pills) of effects of estrogen excess, such as nausea, edema and leg cramps. Other minor side effects include acne, breast discomfort, depression, gastrointestinal upsets, headaches and vaginal infections. More significant but less common side effects include the risks of thrombophlebitis, increased blood pressure, increased blood sugar and gallbladder disease. It is possible that these are slightly decreased in this lower dose. The risk of certain side effects such as heart disease and gallbladder disease appear to increase with age (especially over the age of 35) while a history of true migraine headaches is associated with increased headaches and risk (though small) of stroke.

precautions

A history of thrombophlebitis, blood clots and migraine headaches is usually a relative contraindication to the use of oral contraceptives. For women with other risk factors, such as age over 35, history of heavy smoking, gallbladder disease, diabetes or high blood pressure, use should be weighed carefully against alternate birth control methods.

drug interactions

Several drug interactions have been suggested but none have been well-documented as clinically significant in most cases.

see essays

Hormonal Drugs. Oral Contraceptives.

Norlestrin 1.0

Norlestrin 2.5

generic ingredients	progestogen = norethindrone estrogen = ethinyl estradiol

action and uses One of many combination birth control pills made up of progesterone-like synthetic hormone and an estrogen. The Norlestrin pills contain somewhat greater amounts of both types of hormones than the similar product Loestrin. Norlestrin 2.5 mg, like Ovral and Ortho-Novum, 10 mg, is a "progestagen-dominant" oral contraceptive, which may affect the type of side effects seen (see below). Norlestrin 1.0 has a lower does of progestogen and resembles many other commonly used oral contraceptives. Like most other oral contraceptives, they act to prevent conception by affecting both pituitary control of reproduction as well as acting locally on the lining of the uterus and the cervical mucus and possibly in other ways. When taken regularly, they are very effective contraceptive drugs.

adult dosage In general, one tablet is taken daily (usually at night) on the first cycle, beginning on the 5th day of menstruation and continuing for 21 days. The pill is then discontinued for 7 days and restarted on the 8th day for another 21-day cycle.

adverse effects Compared with some other oral contraceptives, Norlestrin 2.5 may show a slightly higher incidence of increased appetite and weight gain, acne or hair loss, depression, fatigue, and decreased menstrual flow.

With both 2.5 and 1.0 the other common side effects of oral contraceptives may also be seen, including breast changes, gastrointestinal upset, and vaginitis. Less common, but more significant side effects include the risk of thrombophlebitis, increased blood pressure, increased blood sugar or diabetes, and gallbladder disease. The risk of certain side effects such as heart disease and gallbladder disease appear to increase with age (especially over the age of 35) while a history of true migraine headaches is associated with increased headaches and risk of strokes (rare) and a history of heavy smoking is associated with an increased risk of heart attack, particularly at ages greater than 40.

precautions A history of thrombophlebitis, blood clots or migraine headaches is usually a relative contraindication to use of oral contraceptives. For women with other risk factors, such as age over 35, a history of heavy smoking, gallbladder disease, diabetes or high blood pressure, use should be weighed carefully against alternative birth control methods.

drug interactions

Several drug interactions have been suggested but have not been well documented as significant in the majority of cases.

see essays

Hormonal Drugs. Oral Contraceptives.

Novahistine-DH

generic
ingredients

> decongestant = phenylpropanolamine
> cough suppressant = codeine

action and uses

This is a mixture of a decongestant and codeine, which acts to decrease nasal and upper respiratory congestion and also to decrease coughing. This particular cough/cold mixture does not include an antihistamine and is not likely to cause sedation, which may be a useful attribute. Ideally it should be used only when it is necessary to decrease coughing, and this is not often the case since coughing is a useful protective reflex to get rid of secretions.

adult dosage

Two teaspoons every 4-6 hours, not to exceed 4 doses per 24 hours.

adverse effects

The decongestant present may occasionally cause palpitations or pounding of the heart. Several days' use of any compound with codeine can cause constipation. Other side effects are relatively uncommon.

precautions

Elderly people, or those with diabetes, heart trouble or high blood pressure, should always check with their physician since they may require a lower dose. This drug should only be used for a limited time (2-4 days) in most cases.

drug
dependence

The small quantities of codeine present can cause habituation if the drug is taken for prolonged periods.

drug interactions

The decongestant can raise the blood pressure and counteract the effects of several antihypertensive drugs such as Aldomet and Inderal. Codeine can add to the effects of any other sedating drugs.

see essay

Drugs for Coughs and Colds.

Novahistine Expectorant

generic
ingredients

> expectorant = glyceryl guaiacolate
> cough suppressant = codeine
> decongestant = phenylpropanolamine

| action and uses | This elixir is a mixture of a decongestant, a compound to reduce coughing and an expectorant. It is essentially the same as Novahistine-DH except for the added expectorant, and is similar to a wide variety of cough/cold expectorants available. It is not clear whether expectorants, which are thought (but not proven) to increase or liquefy secretions and thus encourage their removal from the lungs, are effective when combined with codeine, which decreases the urge to cough up the secretions. Therefore, this particular mixture should only be used when decreased coughing is desired and when this will not delay the clearing up of the lung problem. |

action and uses   This elixir is a mixture of a decongestant, a compound to reduce coughing and an expectorant. It is essentially the same as Novahistine-DH except for the added expectorant, and is similar to a wide variety of cough/cold expectorants available. It is not clear whether expectorants, which are thought (but not proven) to increase or liquefy secretions and thus encourage their removal from the lungs, are effective when combined with codeine, which decreases the urge to cough up the secretions. Therefore, this particular mixture should only be used when decreased coughing is desired and when this will not delay the clearing up of the lung problem.

adult dosage   Two teaspoons every 4-6 hours, not to exceed 4 doses per 24 hours.

adverse effects   The expectorant may cause some nausea. The decongestant may occasionally cause palpitations or pounding of the heart. Several days' use of any compound containing codeine can cause constipation. Other side effects are uncommon.

precautions   Elderly people, or those with diabetes, heart trouble or high blood pressure, should always check with their physician since they may require a lower dose. The preparation should be used only for limited periods (2-4 days) in most cases.

drug dependence   The small quantities of codeine present can cause habituation if the drug is taken for prolonged periods.

drug interactions   The decongestant can raise the blood pressure and counteract the effects of several antihypertensive drugs such as Aldomet and Inderal. Codeine can add to the effects of any other sedating drugs.

see essay   *Drugs for Coughs and Colds.*

Omnipen (brand name for ampicillin). See AMPICILLIN.

Orinase

generic name

| tolbutamide (available by generic name) |

action and uses   A drug which lowers glucose levels in the blood, used to treat diabetes. Because Orinase can be taken orally (unlike insulin) it is termed an "oral hypoglycemic" drug. It is similar to other oral antidiabetic drugs such as Diabinase and Tolinase, but not DBI. Orinase works by stimulating the pancreas to produce insulin and by helping the cells to use glucose. It is only of value in diabetics who are able to make insulin. Such patients usually have mild diabetes which often becomes evident toward middle age (and is therefore known as maturity onset diabetes). Oral hypoglycemic drugs should only be taken if dietary measures alone have failed to control the condition. Resistance to the effects of Orinase often develops after a few months to years. It is recommended that a withdrawal of oral antidiabetic drugs be tried every six months to one year since their continued use may not be needed. The long term benefits versus risks of this and related drugs are now widely debated.

adult dosage
The dosage is individualized, but is usually 500 mg twice daily, with subsequent adjustment according to response.

adverse effects
The most common and hazardous adverse effect is excessive *lowering* of the blood sugar, which can cause symptoms of dizziness, weakness, cold sweats and mental dullness. Older persons and those on several other drugs (see drug interactions below) or with liver or kidney disease are more prone to this. In proper dosage, other side effects are unusual, but rashes, blood or liver abnormalities and water retention can occur.

precautions
This drug should be avoided by pregnant or potentially pregnant and nursing women, as well as those with significant kidney, or liver disease. Those allergic to sulfa drugs may develop an allergy to this drug.

drug interactions
Thiazide diuretics (as hydrochlorothiazide, Diuril, Hygroton) can aggravate diabetes and may increase the dose requirement of the oral antidiabetic drug. A number of drugs can increase the risk of low blood sugar due to increased levels of drug. These include insulin, sulfa drugs, anti-inflammatory drugs such as aspirin, Butazolidin and Tandearil and the anticonvulsant Dilantin. Inderal (propranolol) can also cause dangerous interactions and disguise the symptoms of hypoglycemia. Alcohol can cause a flushing reaction when taken with this drug.

see essay
Drugs for Diabetes.

Ornade Spansule Capsules

generic ingredients

antihistamine = chlorpheniramine
decongestant = phenylpropanolamine
anticholinergic = isopropamide iodide

action and uses
This mixture of ingredients includes a decongestant, an

antihistamine and an anticholinergic (which causes drying of the secretions), for the relief of symptoms of allergic sinusitis and for severe symptoms of a cold. It is not indicated for asthma.

adult dosage
One Spansule every 12 hours as needed for symptoms.

adverse effects
The most common side effect is drowsiness, due to the antihistamine. Less commonly, there may be excessive dryness of the mouth and nose, palpitations or nervousness. Other side effects are infrequent but more likely to occur in people with heart disease, high blood pressure or prostate trouble.

precautions
This drug should be avoided by pregnant, potentially pregnant and nursing women. Because of the presence of iodide, persons allergic to iodide should not take this drug; for the same reason, prolonged use is not indicated. Caution in driving and operating machinery is necessary if a sedative effect is noticed. Persons taking medicines for high blood pressure or heart ailments should check with their physicians before using Ornade since the decongestant may elevate the blood pressure.

drug interactions
The sedative effect of the antihistamine can be additive to alcohol and other sedatives and tranquilizers. The decongestant can raise the blood pressure and thus counteract the effects of some antihypertensive drugs. The anticholinergic drug can also be additive in its effect on certain antispasmodic drugs used for treatment of ulcer or bladder dysfunctions (such as Pro-Banthine) or can interact with tricyclic antidepressant drugs (such as Elavil). The iodide in the compound can interfere with certain tests of thyroid function.

see essay
Drugs for Coughs and Colds.

Ortho-Novum

generic
ingredients

| progestogen = norethindrone |
| estrogen = mestranol |

action and uses
Ortho-Novum is one of many combination birth control pills containing a progesterone-like synthetic hormone and estrogen. It acts like most other birth control pills to prevent contraception by affecting pituitary control of reproduction as well as acting locally on the lining of the uterus and the cervical mucus, and possibly in other ways. It has a higher dose of both the progestogen and the estrogen than the other Ortho-Novum preparations (1/50

and 1/80) and is generally used less frequently because of this. It is essentially identical to Norinyl 2 mg. When taken regularly, it is a highly effective oral contraceptive drug.

adult dosage

In general, one tablet is taken daily (usually at night) on the first cycle, beginning on the 5th day of menstruation and continuing for 21 days. The pill is then discontinued for 7 days and restarted on the 8th day for another 21-day cycle.

adverse effects

Like all oral contraceptives, a variety of side effects may occur including weight gain, increased appetite, depression or fatigue, breast changes, gastrointestinal upset, headache, and increased vaginal discharge or infection. More significant but less common side effects include the risk of thrombophlebitis, increased blood pressure, increased blood sugar and gallbladder disease. The risk of certain side effects such as heart disease and gallbladder disease appears to increase with age (especially over the age of 35) while a history of true migraine headaches is associated with increased headaches and risk (though small) of actual strokes.

precautions

A history of thrombophlebitis, blood clots and migraine headaches is usually a relative contraindication to the use of oral contraceptives. For women with other risk factors, such as age over 35, history of heavy smoking, gallbladder disease, diabetes or high blood pressure, use should be weighed carefully against alternative birth control methods.

drug interactions

Several drug interactions have been suggested but none have been well-documented as clinically significant in most cases.

see essays

Hormonal Drugs. Oral Contraceptives.

Ortho-Novum 1/50

generic ingredients

progestogen = norethindrone
estrogen = mestranol

action and uses

Ortho-Novum 1/50, which is essentially identical to Norinyl 1/50, is a combination of a progesterone-like hormone and an estrogen, and contains the same dose (50 micrograms) of estrogen. Recent studies have suggested that lowering the dose of estrogen may be associated with a lower incidence of estrogen-related side effects, although the incidence of breakthrough bleeding and spotting tends to be increased, especially in earlier cycles. It acts like most birth control pills to prevent contraception by affecting the pituitary control of reproduction, as well as acting locally on the lining of the uterus and the cervical mucus, and possibly in other ways. When taken regularly it is a very effective contraceptive drug.

adult dosage

In general one tablet is taken daily (usually at night) on the first cycle, beginning on the 5th day of menstruation and continuing for 21 days. The pills are then discontinued for 7 days and restarted on the 8th day for another 21-day cycle.

adverse effects

Use of oral contraception pills has been associated with a variety of side effects. Ortho-Novum 1/50 (as well as Norinyl 1/50) may be associated with a higher incidence of breakthrough bleeding or spotting, but there appears to be a slightly decreased incidence (as compared with some other higher estrogen pills) of effects of estrogen excess, such as nausea, edema and leg cramps. Other minor side effects include acne, breast discomfort, depression, gastrointestinal upsets, headaches and vaginal infections. More significant but less common side effects include the risks of thrombophlebitis, increased blood pressure, increased blood sugar and gallbladder disease. It is possible that these are slightly decreased in this lower dose. The risk of certain side effects such as heart disease and gallbladder disease appears to increase with age (especially over the age of 35) while a history of true migraine headaches is associated with increased headaches and risk (although small) of stroke.

precautions

A history of thrombophlebitis, blood clots and migraine headaches is usually a relative contraindication to the use of oral contraceptives. For women with other risk factors, such as age over 35, history of heavy smoking, gallbladder disease, diabetes or high blood pressure, use should be weighed carefully against alternative birth control methods.

drug interactions

Several drug interactions have been suggested but none have been well-documented as clinically significant in most cases.

see essays

Hormonal Drugs. Oral Contraceptives.

Ortho-Novum 1/80

generic
ingredients

progestogen = norethindrone estrogen = mestranol

action and uses	Ortho-Novum 1/80 is one of the four Ortho-Novum oral contraceptives combining a progesterone-like synthetic hormone with an estrogen. It has a lower dose of both the progestogen and the estrogen than plain Ortho-Novum but a higher dose of estrogen than Ortho-Novum 1/50. It is sometimes used when breakthrough bleeding with a lower dose of estrogen in Ortho-Novum 1/50 occurs. The product is essentially identical to Norinyl 1/80. It acts like most other oral contraceptives to affect pituitary control of reproduction as well as locally on the lining of the uterus and the cervical mucus, and possibly in other ways. When taken regularly, it is a very effective contraceptive drug.
adult dosage	In general, one tablet is taken daily (usually at night) on the first cycle, beginning on the 5th day of menstruation and continuing for 21 days. The pill is then discontinued for 7 days and restarted on the 8th day for another 21-day cycle.
adverse effects	Like all oral contraceptives, a variety of side effects may occur including weight gain, increased appetite, depression or fatigue, breast changes, gastrointestinal upset, headache, and increased vaginal discharge or infection. More significant but less common side effects include the risk of thrombophlebitis, increased blood pressure, increased blood sugar and gallbladder disease. The risk of certain side effects such as heart disease and gallbladder disease appears to increase with age (especially over the age of 35) while a history of true migraine headaches is associated with increased headaches and risk (though small) of stroke.
precautions	A history of thrombophlebitis, blood clots and migraine headaches is usually a relative contraindication to the use of oral contraceptives. For women with other risk factors, such as age over 35, history of heavy smoking, gallbladder disease, diabetes or high blood pressure, use should be weighed carefully against alternative birth control methods.
drug interactions	Several drug interactions have been suggested but none have been well-documented as clinically significant in most cases.
see essays	*Hormonal Drugs. Oral Contraceptives.*

Ovral

generic ingredients	progestogen = norgestrel estrogen = ethinyl estradiol

action and uses

Ovral is one of many combination birth control pills made up of a progesterone-like synthetic hormone and an estrogen. Ovral contains somewhat greater amounts of hormones than the similar product, Lo Ovral. Norgestrel is believed to be a somewhat more potent progesterone-like hormone so that Ovral, like Norlestrin 2.5 mg and Ortho-Novum 2 mg, is a "progestogen-dominant" oral contraceptive, which may affect the type of side effects seen (see below). Like most other oral contraceptives, it acts to prevent conception by affecting pituitary control of reproduction as well as acting locally on the lining of the uterus and the cervical mucus and possibly in other ways. When taken regularly like all oral contraceptives, it is a very effective contraceptive drug.

adult dosage

In general, one tablet is taken daily (usually at night) on the first cycle, beginning on the 5th day of menstruation and continuing for 21 days. The pill is then discontinued for 7 days and restarted on the 8th day for another 21-day cycle.

adverse effects

Compared with some other oral contraceptives, Ovral may produce a slightly higher incidence of increased appetite and weight gain, acne or hair loss, depression, fatigue and decreased menstrual flow.

The other more common side effects of oral contraceptives may also be seen, including breast changes, gastrointestinal upset, and vaginitis. Less common but more significant side effects include the risk of thrombophlebitis, increased blood pressure, increased blood sugar or diabetes, and gallbladder disease. The risk of certain side effects such as heart disease and gallbladder disease appears to increase with age (especially over the age of 35) while a history of true migraine headaches is associated with increased headaches and risk of strokes (rare), and a history of heavy smoking is associated with an increased risk of heart attack, particularly in women of 40 and over.

precautions

A history of thrombophlebitis, blood clots or migraine headaches is usually a relative contraindication to use of oral contraceptives. For women with other risk factors, such as age over 35, a history of heavy smoking, gallbladder disease, diabetes or high blood pressure, use should be weighed carefully against alternative birth control methods.

drug interactions Several drug interactions have been suggested but have not been well documented as significant in the majority of cases.

see essays *Hormonal Drugs. Oral Contraceptives.*

Ovral-28

generic ingredients

progestogen = norgestrel estrogen = ethinyl estradiol

Ovral-28 is one of many combination birth control pills made up of a progesterone-like synthetic hormone and an estrogen. It is essentially identical to Ovral except that it is packaged with 21 combination pills and seven "dummy" pills so that one pill is taken each day during the month, which maintains the cycle. This form is sometimes useful for those who tend to get confused or who vary in their cycle. The remainder of the description is identical to that under Ovral.

Ovulen

generic ingredients

progestogen = ethynodiol diacetate estrogen = ethinyl estradiol

action and uses Ovulen is one of many combination birth control pills containing a progesterone-like drug and an estrogen. It acts like most other oral contraceptives to prevent conception by affecting pituitary control of reproduction as well as acting locally on the lining of the uterus and the cervical mucus, and possibly in other ways. When taken regularly, like all oral contraceptives, it is a very effective contraceptive drug. It is similar to Demulen.

adult dosage In general, one tablet is taken daily (usually at night) on the first cycle, beginning on the 5th day of menstruation and continuing for 21 days. The pill is then discontinued for 7 days and restarted on the 8th day for another 21-day cycle.

adverse effects Like all oral contraceptives, a variety of side effects may occur, including weight gain, increased appetite, depression or fatigue, breast changes, gastrointestinal upset, headache, and increased vaginal discharge or infection.

More significant but less common side effects include the risk of thrombophlebitis, increased blood pressure, increased blood sugar and gallbladder disease. The risk of certain side effects such as heart disease and gallbladder disease appears to increase with age (especially over the age of 35) while history of true migraine headaches is associated with increased headaches and risk (though small) of stroke.

precautions A history of thrombophlebitis, blood clots and migraine headaches is usually a relative contraindication to the use of oral contraceptives. For women with other risk factors, such as age over 35, history of heavy smoking, gallbladder disease, diabetes or high blood pressure, use should be weighed carefully against alternative birth control methods.

drug interactions Several drug interactions have been suggested but none have been well-documented as significant in most cases.

see essays *Hormonal Drugs. Oral Contraceptives.*

Papaverine (generic name). See PAVABID.

Parafon Forte

generic
ingredients

muscle relaxant = chlorzoxazone	
pain reliever = acetaminophen	

action and uses Parafon Forte is a combination drug used to treat various types of muscle spasm, most commonly experienced in back or neck strain. It is a combination of the mild pain reliever acetaminophen (Tylenol, Nebs) with a drug which is believed to act on the spinal cord to inhibit local muscle spasm and thus relieve discomfort. This "muscle relaxing" drug, chlorzoxazone, is also used alone as the drug Paraflex.

adult dosage One or two tablets, 3-4 times per day, adjusted according to need.

adverse effects Occasional gastrointestinal upset or drowsiness and dizziness may occur. Rarely, liver abnormalities have been reported to occur with chlorzoxazone. Some persons may also have reddish-purple urine which is not thought to present a problem.

precautions Parafon Forte may cause drowsiness and therefore presents a hazard in driving or operating machinery. The drug should be avoided by pregnant, potentially pregnant and nursing women.

drug interactions	Since both ingredients in this combination have been reported to cause liver damage in excessive doses, the possibility of their interaction to increase this effect is a possibility.
see essay	*Non-Narcotic Pain Relievers.*

Paregoric (camphorated tincture of opium)

action and uses	A preparation used to treat diarrhea. It contains only a minute amount of morphine (0.04%) but, because of morphine's pronounced constipating effect on the intestinal tract, even this small amount is enough to make paregoric an effective remedy for simple diarrhea. Paregoric is often combined with kaolin and pectin to enhance its antidiarrheal action. Among the products containing this combination are Parepectolin, Ka-Pek with Paregoric, Kaoparin with Paregoric, and Dia-Quel. Although Paregoric is effective, some authorities feel that prolonged use may lengthen the illness by allowing retention of bacteria or toxins in the bowel.
adult dosage	Usually 1-2 teaspoons 1-4 times per day for no more than 2 days.
adverse effects	Side effects with paregoric are few, although those persons who are allergic to morphine may also be allergic to this drug. One minor side effect, ironically, is constipation, which may result if the paregoric is continued too long after the diarrhea stops.
precautions	If diarrhea persists for more then 2-3 days, its cause should be investigated. Paregoric should be kept in an amber bottle away from extreme heat and should be thrown away after five years.
drug dependence	Psychological and/or physical dependence can potentially result if this drug is taken in large doses over an extended period.
drug interactions	Oversedation might result from mixing paregoric with sedatives, sleeping pills, tranquilizers, or alcohol.
see essay	*Drugs for Diarrhea.*

Pavabid

generic name	papaverine (available by generic name)

action and uses	This drug is promoted and used for disorders causing decreased circulation to the brain, feet or hands. Although

it relaxes blood vessels (and therefore increases the flow of blood) when injected directly into the vessels in normal persons. There is no clear evidence that, taken orally, it can increase blood flow in abnormal states, such as when there is arteriosclerosis (fatty obstruction) of the blood vessels, or when a person experiences coldness of the extremities or pain with exercise (intermittent claudication). It is also used, but is questionably effective, in conditions where there is temporary spasm of the arteries, such as Raynaud's phenomenon.

adult dosage 100-150 mg 2 to 3 times a day.

adverse effects Pavabid is well tolerated, but may cause various gastrointestinal reactions as well as dizziness, especially with rapid change in position, and rapid heart rate. Allergic rashes may also occur, and rarely, liver abnormalities.

precautions This drug should not be used directly after minor or major surgery or childbirth. It should be avoided in pregnant, potentially pregnant or nursing women as well as those with ulcers.

drug interactions Pavabid may add to effects of other more effective blood-vessel relaxing drugs, such as nitroglycerin or Apresoline, to lower blood pressure.

see essay *Drugs Used to Prevent or Treat Circulation Disorders.*

Pediamycin

generic name

erythromycin ethyl succinate (available by generic name)

action and uses A commonly used antibiotic which comes from the mold *Streptomyces*. It acts on bacteria to inhibit production of proteins but has no effect on human cells. Pediamycin (erythromycin) is most commonly used in mild to moderate infections where penicillin is indicated but allergy is present. These infections include bacterial sore throat ("strep throat"), respiratory or lung infections and some venereal diseases. It is seldom used in very serious infections.

adult dosage The usual adult dosage is 250 to 500 mg every six hours, preferably on an empty stomach. Pediamycin comes in several forms which are suitable for administration to children. Dosage must be determined by the physician.

adverse effects The most frequent side effect is gastrointestinal upset, including nausea, belching and diarrhea. Rashes and other allergic reactions can occur but are not as frequent as with other antibiotics.

This antibiotic, like all others, should be taken for the time period directed, and every dose should be taken. Failure to do this can result in inadequate treatment of the infection, recurrence, or development of a resistant infection. Pediamycin should be used with caution by pregnant, potentially pregnant and nursing women.

drug interactions

Erythromycin may interfere with the effectiveness of penicillin and Cleocin.

see essay

Drugs to Treat Infections.

Penicillin G

trade names

Pentids, Pfizerpen

action and uses

One of the most important of all the antibiotics and the prototype for the group of penicillin drugs. It is produced by the bread mold *penicillium* and purified for use in tablets and for injection. Penicillin G acts to prevent formation of the cell walls of bacteria. This prevents their growth and multiplication. There is no effect on human cells due to differences in structure. Penicillin G is most effective against the group of bacteria which commonly cause sore throats ("strep throat"), and certain abcesses, although some bacteria in abcesses (staphylococcal or "staph") can become resistant to penicillin G, especially in hospitals. Penicillin G is also effective against syphilis and gonorrhea in most cases, although these venereal diseases are often treated with long-acting injections of penicillin G (Bicillin). Penicillin is not as effective for treatment of serious infections by the group of bacteria called Gram negative bacilli, which cause infections in the urinary tract, bowel and elsewhere. Penicillin G has no effect on virus or fungal infections.

adult dosage

The dose varies according to the infection. When given by injection, the dose may range from 0.6-1.2 to 4.8 million units every 4 to 6 hours, depending on the need. Penicillin G taken orally tends to be destroyed by stomach acid and food tends to interfere with its entry into the body so although available it is not used as frequently as penicillin V.

adverse effects

If taken orally, the most common adverse effect is gastrointestinal upset, cramps, or diarrhea. Given by injections or orally, the primary concern is the occurrence of allergic reactions, which can include skin rashes or hives, swelling of the face or throat, difficulty breathing, or some time later, joint pains and fever.

precautions   Penicillin G should not be taken when there is known allergy to any of the penicillin drugs. Nursing mothers should check with the physician. Penicillin G, like all antibiotics, should be taken for the entire time period directed (usually 5-10 days) even though symptoms may disappear. Otherwise infections may recur and even develop resistance to the antibiotic.

drug interactions   In some cases, the effect of penicillin may be decreased if erythromycin or chloramphenicol is also taken.

see essay   *Drugs to Treat Infections.*

Penicillin V (generic name). See V-CILLIN K.

Penicillin VK

generic name

> phenoxymethyl penicillin (available by generic name)

action and uses   A semi-synthetic penicillin antibiotic which is almost identical to penicillin G in its action and adverse effects except that due to a small difference in its chemical structure, it is more effective orally. This is because it is not easily destroyed by stomach acid. See the discussion of Penicillin G, above.

adult dosage   The usual oral dose is 250-500 gm (equivalent to 0.4-0.8 million units) every 6 hours on an empty stomach, but this is individualized, according to the infection. Once a course of Penicillin VK is prescribed, it should be taken for the prescribed length of time (usually 5-10 days) even though symptoms may disappear. This is very important since the infection may otherwise recur and even develop resistance to the antibiotic.

Pentids

generic name

> penicillin G (available by generic name)

action and uses   The action and uses are the same as those recorded for Penicillin G, described above.

Pentobarbital (generic name). See NEMBUTAL.

Pen-Vee-K

generic name

> phenoxymethyl penicillin (available by generic name)

action and uses
A semi-synthetic penicillin antibiotic which is almost identical to penicillin G in its action and adverse effects except that due to a small difference in its chemical structure, it is more effective orally. This is because it is not easily destroyed by stomach acid. See the discussion of Penicillin G, above.

adult dosage
The usual oral dose is 250-500 mg (equivalent of 0.4-0.8 million units) every six hours on an empty stomach, but this is individualized, according to the infection.

Percodan

generic ingredients

> narcotic pain reliever = oxycodone
> pain relievers = aspirin,
> phenacetin
> mild stimulant = caffeine

action and uses
A strong pain reliever used in the treatment of severe pain. It combines the narcotic analgesic oxycodone, a chemical relative of codeine, with the non-narcotic analgesics aspirin and phenacetin and the mild stimulant caffeine. Oxycodone is slightly stronger than codeine and by itself would be a useful alternative narcotic for moderate to severe pain. Prescriptions for this drug are specially controlled because of the hazard of abuse.

adult dosage
Usually 1-2 tablets every 4-6 hours as needed for pain.

adverse effects
The oxycodone in Percodan, can like codeine, cause nausea and constipation, and occasional allergic reactions. The aspirin in the preparation can cause stomach irritation and bleeding. The phenacetin can cause kidney damage.

precautions
Percodan should be taken with caution by patients with stomach disorders or impaired kidney function if prolonged use is necessary. Pregnant or potentially pregnant or nursing mothers should avoid this drug if possible.

drug dependence
Percodan can cause psychological and/or physical dependence or addiction if used for extended periods of time.

drug interactions
Oversedation may result when Percodan is taken concurrently with alcohol, tranquilizers, sedatives, sleeping pills, antidepressants, and antihistamines. The aspirin adds to the effects of oral anticoagulants, increasing the risk of

bleeding, and to the effects of cortisone-like drugs, increasing the risk of peptic ulcer.

see essay *Narcotic Pain Relievers.*

Periactin

generic name

cyproheptadine

action and uses
An antihistamine drug which differs somewhat from other antihistamines in that it also blocks another substance in the body called serotonin. It is most commonly used as an antihistamine for treatment of allergic dermatitis and other allergy problems. However, because of its antiserotonin effect it can also be used to treat the diarrhea which occurs in patients who have had their stomachs removed (called "dumping syndrome") and in patients with a special kind of tumor called carcinoid (a tumor which produces a serotonin and causes severe diarrhea and flushing).

adult dosage
The usual dose for treatment of allergic condition is 4 mg 3 to 4 times per day. Somewhat higher doses are sometimes used for treatment of the special kinds of diarrhea mentioned above.

adverse effects
Periactin shares the ability of antihistamines to cause drowsiness in some, and sometimes other effects such as dry mouth and stomach distress. It differs in that it has been shown to cause weight gain with long use in some patients.

precautions
This drug may interfere with driving or operating machinery. It should be avoided by pregnant or potentially pregnant women and nursing mothers.

drug interactions
Periactin is additive to other sedative and tranquilizer drugs such as sleeping pills and alcohol. It is also additive to strong antispasmodic drugs of the kind used to treat stomach problems, such as Pro-Banthine and Librax, as well as tricyclic antidepressants such as Elavil.

see essay *Antihistamines.*

Phenaphen with Codeine

generic ingredients

narcotic = codeine
pain reliever = acetaminophen

action and uses
A popular, mild analgesic drug available with and without the addition of codeine, a narcotic analgesic. With codeine it is used to treat more severe pain than can be relieved by

simple analgesics such as aspirin or acetaminophen.

adult dosage
One to two tablets every 4-6 hours as needed for pain.

adverse effects
The major side effects which can occur are due to the codeine, which can cause constipation, occasional nausea and vomiting, and occasionally dizziness. Large doses or acetaminophen can cause serious liver disease.

precautions
Because habitual use is a hazard, the forms containing codeine should be used only when non-narcotic analgesics are not effective.

drug dependence
Prolonged use of codeine may cause dependence.

drug interactions
The codeine effect can be additive to other narcotic drugs as well as to other sedating drugs such as tranquilizers or alcohol.

see essay
Narcotic Pain Relievers.

Phenazopyridine (generic name). See PYRIDIUM.

Phenergan Expectorant

generic Ingredients

antihistamine = promethazine
expectorants = potassium guaiacol-sulfonate,
            sodium citrate, citric acid
miscellaneous = ipecac, alcohol

Phenergan Expectorant with Codeine
Phenergan VC Expectorant

generic ingredients

decongestant = phenylephrine
antihistamine = promethazine
expectorants = potassium guaiacol-sulfonate,
            sodium citrate, citric acid
miscellaneous = ipecac, alcohol

Phenergan VC Expectorant with Codeine

generic ingredients

generic ingredients are the same as Phenergan VC Expectorant except for addition of the narcotic cough-suppressant, codeine.

action and uses
These are mixtures of ingredients for relief of upper respiratory symptoms, nasal congestion (the antihistamine and decongestant) and for promoting liquefication (the expectorant) and elimination of dried secretions. They are

used for relief of symptoms of colds and some allergies, but not asthma. Whether these compounds are actually useful as expectorants is not known, since it has been difficult to test the expectorants for their effectiveness. Phenergan VC Expectorant differs from Phenergan Expectorant only in the addition of the decongestant, phenylephrine. Both are available with or without the cough-suppressant narcotic, codeine, which should be used only when cough suppression is really needed.

adult dosage
One to two teaspoons every 4-6 hours as needed for the relief of symptoms.

adverse effects
Phenergan may occasionally cause drowsiness and the expectorant may cause nausea in some cases. The codeine preparations may cause constipation and also nausea. The decongestant in the VC preparations may cause palpitations or nervousness, and a lower dose may be required in those with heart disease, high blood pressure or diabetes. This drug should be avoided by pregnant or potentially pregnant women and nursing mothers.

precautions
If sedation is an effect, then driving or operating machinery can be hazardous. Persons with high blood pressure should not take the Phenergan VC Expectorant.

drug dependence
Although the dose is small, prolonged use of large doses of the codeine-containing compounds can cause habituation.

drug interactions
The sedative effect of Phenergan and codeine can be additive to alcohol or tranquilizing drugs. The alcohol in the mixture can cause reactions in persons taking Antabuse or Flagyl. The decongestant can counteract the effect of drugs used to treat high blood pressure.

see essays
Drugs for Coughs and Colds. Antihistamines.

Phenobarbital

brand name

Luminal

action and uses
A widely-used drug for the treatment of anxiety, seizures (such as epileptic seizures), and insomnia. Phenobarbital is one of the group of drugs known as barbiturates. It has been used for many years both as a tranquilizer and to treat seizures. In the last 15 years, with the introduction of newer tranquilizers such as diazepam (Valium) and meprobamate (Miltown and Equanil), its use as a tranquilizer has decreased, but it is still a major anticonvulsant or anti-epileptic drug. Sometimes it is used in combination

with other anticonvulsant drugs, such as Dilantin. Phenobarbital is incorporated into more than 50 combination products which are used for treating illness ranging from stomach ulcers to asthma, since the questionable assumption is made that many of these conditions are associated with anxiety.

adult dosage For treatment of anxiety, usually 15-30 mg, 2 to 3 times per day. For sleep, usually 60-100 mg at bedtime. For prevention of seizures 30-90 mg may be given once daily since it stays in the body for more than a day.

adverse effects When phenobarbital is used as a sleeping pill it may cause a "hangover" effect the following morning. It may also cause a feeling of depression and tiredness, or infrequently nausea, vomiting, and diarrhea. Allergic reactions, such as skin rashes, may also occur.

drug dependence If used for longer than 7 to 10 days, "tolerance" to phenobarbital may develop, which means that a larger dose will be needed to produce the same tranquilizing effect. If this occurs dependence on the drug may develop and if it is suddenly discontinued there may be withdrawal symptoms such as anxiety, insomnia, or even seizures (if the dose is large or if a seizure disorder is present). Therefore, it must be stopped slowly after being used for a long time.

precautions Phenobarbital and other barbiturates have long been a major cause of suicidal and accidental drug overdose and death. If taken in high doses they can be very dangerous and lethal. They can be hazardous if taken with alcohol or other tranquilizers.

drug interactions Phenobarbital can interact with many other drugs, particularly the anticoagulant Coumadin, to decrease its effect and increase the risk of clotting.

Its effect is additive to the effects of other tranquilizers, sleeping pills and alcohol. The combination with any of these drugs can be very hazardous, causing suppression of breathing and even death.

see essays *Sleeping Pills. Minor Tranquilizers. Drugs for Seizures or Convulsions.*

Phenoxymethylpenicillin (generic name). See PENICILLIN VK, V-CILLIN K, PEN-VEE-K.

Phentermine resin (generic name). See IONAMIN.

Phenylbutazone (generic name). See BUTAZOLIDIN.

Pilocarpine (generic name). See ISOPTO-CARPINE.

Placidyl

generic name

> ethchlorvynol

action and uses
A nighttime sedative or sleeping pill. In chemical makeup, it differs from other sleeping pills, though its effects are similar.

adult dosage
Usually 50 mg at bedtime. Once taken, its sleep-inducing effects are felt within 15-45 minutes, and last for 5-6 hours.

adverse effects
Like most other sleeping pills and sedatives, Placidyl can cause dizziness, headache and morning hangover. Unlike other sleeping pills and sedatives, it has occasionally produced permanent changes in vision and possible changes in nerve function, when used over an extended period of time. The possibility of these adverse effects tend to make its use, especially for more than a few days, questionable.

precautions
Placidyl should not be taken by pregnant or potentially pregnant women or nursing mothers; nor by patients with neurological or eye disease. It may also interfere with driving or operating machinery.

drug dependence
Psychological and/or physical dependence are possible with extended use of this drug, and withdrawal symptoms occur when it is suddenly stopped after being used for some time.

drug interactions
Placidyl's sedative effects can be increased by alcohol, other sedatives or sleeping pills, tranquilizers, antihistamines and pain relievers. It is especially hazardous in combination with any of the tricyclic antidepressants (such as Flagyl, Tofranil and Sinequan). Placidyl can decrease the effect of anticoagulants, such as Coumadin, thus increasing the possibility of clotting.

see essay
Sleeping Pills.

Polaramine

generic name

> dexchlorpheniramine (available by generic name)

action and uses
A commonly prescribed antihistamine which is frequently used to treat allergic conditions, especially allergic rhinitis, sinusitis, or conjunctivitis (redness of the eye). It shares the effects of most other antihistamines by blocking the effects of histamine and thus can decrease itching of the skin due to allergies, hives or rashes. It also can sometimes

have a sedating effect, although it is not customarily used for this. It is not useful for treatment of asthma. It is usually much less expensive in generic form, or, as chlorpheniramine.

adult dosage

Polaramine is available in oral tablets and liquid forms. The usual oral dose is 2 mg 2 to 4 times daily or one 6 mg Repetab twice daily as needed for treatment of allergic conditions.

adverse effects

Although possibly less frequently than with some other antihistamines, Polaramine may cause significant sedation in some people. Other side effects are relatively rare, but can include dry mouth, blurred vision, or difficulty in urinating, especially in older persons or those with glaucoma or prostate trouble.

precautions

The sedative effects may interfere with driving or operating machinery. This drug should be used with caution in those with glaucoma or prostate trouble. It should also be avoided by pregnant or potentially pregnant women and nursing mothers.

drug interactions

Polaramine is additive to other sedative or tranquilizing drugs and alcohol. It is also additive to other antispasmodic drugs used to treat ulcers or stomach problems, such as Pro-Banthine or Librax, to cause excessive dry mouth, constipation and difficulty in urinating.

see essay

Antihistamines.

Polycillin (brand name for ampicillin). See AMPICILLIN.

Poly-Vi-Flor

generic ingredients

vitamins = A, D, C, E, B complex, folic acid mineral = fluoride

action and uses

A fixed combination vitamin-mineral supplement used for children. The vitamins are used to supplement the regular food of infants and children. The fluoride is used to help prevent dental cavities, when there is no fluoride in the water supply.

adult dosage

One tablet daily of the chewable tablets.

adverse effects

Both vitamins A and D can cause serious adverse effects if taken in excess. Vitamin A can cause liver and skin abnormalities, vitamin D, bone abnormalities.

precautions

Poly-Vi-Flor should not be used if the local community water already contains fluoride. Only the dose recommended should be used, preferably with a doctor's advice.

drug interactions | No significant interactions occur at the recommended dose.

see essay | *Vitamins and Minerals.*

Potassium (generic name). See SLOW-K.

Potassium Chloride

trade names

Kaochlor, Kaon-Cl, Kato, Kayciel, KEFF, K-Lor, Klorvess, K/Lyte/Cl, Kolyum, Pfiklor, Rum-K, Slow-K.

action and uses | This is a mineral salt that is essential to the body's function and is usually given to replace the body potassium lost from the kidneys. The loss is most often caused by diuretics ("water pills") or cortisone-like drugs, but can also occur in some diseases. Thus, it forms a common part of a regimen for high blood pressure or heart failure. Potassium is vital to the body's function, and excessive loss can cause muscle weakness, tiredness, and dizziness, and when severe, can be life-threatening.

Potassium is present in many foods, especially fruits such as oranges, melons, dried fruits, and vegetables such as tomatoes and potatoes. If the amounts needed are small, they may be replaced in the diet, or by use of salt substitutes, such as Lite-salt, which also contain this mineral. If larger amounts are required, as determined by checking the blood level of potassium, it is necessary to give potassium orally. This has been a major problem, since potassium chloride, the only form of potassium which is really effective, is very distasteful to many persons. It commonly comes, in the much less expensive generic form, as a liquid with or without various flavorings. It also comes in a variety of trade-name preparations as powders or liquids. Many of these are more palatable, but they are also much more costly, and many contain other forms of potassium, such as potassium citrate, which are not as effective. It is the amount of potassium *chloride* taken which is important. The pill form of potassium chloride, Slow-K, is discussed under that name.

adult dosage | This varies with need but is most often 40-80 milliequivalents per day. It can be taken with juice or food to disguise the taste.

adverse effects | The most common adverse effect of potassium is its metallic bitter taste on the tongue. Also common is stomach irritation or nausea, which can be avoided by diluting the mineral (in concentrated form, it is very irritating). Rarely, ulceration of the stomach or bowel can occur if the potassium is concentrated in one area. If excess potassium is used in the presence of kidney failure, serious effects on the heart can occur.

precautions

Potassium should be used only with special instructions, and occasional blood tests if it must be given with severe kidney disease or with potassium-retaining diuretics.

drug interactions

If given with potassium-retaining diuretics such as Dyazide, Dyrenium, Aldactone or Aldactezide, potassium preparations can cause dangerously high levels of potassium in the blood.

see essay

Vitamins and Minerals.

Prednisone

trade names

Deltasone, Meticorten, Orasone

action and uses

Prednisone is one of several drugs referred to as "steroids" or "corticosteroids." Corticosteroids are hormones produced by the cortex of the adrenal glands. Drugs with very similar properties to these hormones can also be made by chemical synthesis. Prednisone is one of these "synthetic" steroid hormones, and is the most commonly used corticosteroid. Prednisone is used in a wide variety of disorders in two major ways: (1) in small doses it is used to replace the normally present corticosteroid hormones when the adrenal glands are removed or nonfunctional due to disease (Addison's disease); (2) in larger doses it is used to prevent or treat a variety of disorders usually associated with severe inflammation and/or destruction of tissue, such as acute arthritis or serious allergic reactions, as in severe asthma.

Prednisone and related corticosteroids act on many cells in the body to change the production of proteins and the ways in which cells handle carbohydrates and fats, and certain minerals. This promotes several desirable effects when the drug is given in higher doses. First, it acts to suppress inflammation, which can be useful in certain types of arthritis (although it is used as a last resort in this situation); in inflammatory disease of the bowel, such as ulcerative colitis; and in a large variety of skin diseases where there is inflammation of the skin, such as psoriasis, or eczema. Secondly, it acts to suppress certain types of white blood cells and lowers the body's immunity, which can be useful in the treatment of certain types of "auto-immune" diseases (where the body reacts to its own tissues) such as lupus erythematosus, certain types of leukemia where there is an overproduction of the white blood cells as well as in the prevention of rejection of transplanted organs. Thirdly, it acts to inhibit allergic reactions in severe allergic conditions such as asthma, and serious skin allergies such as poison oak and poison ivy. Prednisone has a variety of other actions which are sometimes used in treatment, but more often cause adverse effects as noted below.

adult dosage

The dose is highly individualized and may be as high as 100 mg or more a day, or as little as 5 mg per day. When first started, it is often taken in high doses, sometimes several times a day but when taken chronically, it is usually taken once daily in the morning, or once every other day, depending on the circumstances.

adverse effects

The adverse effects of prednisone are related to both the dose and the length of time the drug is taken. A single dose of any amount of prednisone may usually be taken without significant adverse effects. However, the incidence of serious adverse effects increases considerably with time at any dose greater than the physiological equivalent (approximately 7.5 mg per day). The most common adverse reaction observed in a large series of hospitalized patients on prednisone included disturbances of water and salt to produce edema (or water retention) and loss of potassium (which can cause weakness).

Other common side effects include development of abnormal fat deposits around the face ("moon face"), neck ("buffalo hump") or abodomen, weight gain, increased bruising, gastrointestinal bleeding, and/or upset, and mental confusion, and diabetes. Antacids are frequently given to prevent the gastrointestinal problems. A continuing effect is the decreased susceptibility to infections and often the masking of the symptoms of these infections. For this reason, those with a history of, or exposure to chronic infections such as tuberculosis are observed carefully. With longer use, there is often gradual degeneration of bone and muscle which can cause fractures and muscle weakness, and cataracts may develop. Obviously the use of this drug for long periods requires very careful analysis of benefits versus risks. It has been found that certain, but not all, chronic ailments which require this drug for very long periods can be controlled by giving prednisone every other day. This is desirable whenever possible since it tends to eliminate most of the severe side effects.

Another practical effect of using prednisone relates to the fact that it tends to suppress the normal effect of the adrenal gland. In stress, the adrenal gland puts out much more corticosteroid to help the body handle the stress. The absence of this extra reserve can be life threatening. A person on prednisone does not have this reserve, so that if an accident occurs, or surgery is required, higher doses may be needed for a few days.

precautions Use of prednisone, especially for more than seven days, requires the careful supervision of a physician who should be notified of any changes which occur, especially after altering the dose, or adding any other drug. Persons taking prednisone for long periods should carry a card or wear a bracelet giving this information in the event of an emergency.

drug interactions Prednisone interacts additively with many diuretics such as hydrochlorothiazide or Lasix, to cause excessive loss of potassium, which can cause weakness. Since diuretics are often used to treat the edema caused by corticosteroids, this interaction can be anticipated and prevented by supplementing the potassium intake. Since aspirin and several other anti-inflammatory drugs, such as Motrin, used to treat arthritis, also cause gastric upset and ulcer, they may be additive to this effect of prednisone.

see essay *Steroids or Cortisone-like Drugs.*

Premarin

generic name

conjugated estrogen

action and uses Premarin, whose name is a contraction of "pregnant mare's urine," is a mixture of estrogen female hormone compounds like those found in the horse's urine. In 1976, it was the second most frequently prescribed drug in the United States. It is usually prescribed to replace deficient estrogen due to surgical removal of the ovaries (a natural source of estrogens) or decreased function of the ovaries which occurs in menopause. Premarin is also used in some other types of menstrual dysfunction, in treatment of breast swelling after child delivery, and in the treatment of certain cases of cancer of the prostate in men and of the breast in women.

In the normal premenopausal state, the levels of

estrogens produced by the ovaries fluctuate during the menstrual cycle and along with the other female hormone progesterone, control the menstrual cycle. Estrogens also act on and partly maintain the so-called secondary sex characteristics, including the breasts, the reproductive organs and to a certain extent, hair and fat distribution. They also are believed to affect the skin, bone metabolism and brain function to some extent, as well as other metabolic functions.

With onset of menopause, the amount of estrogen produced by the ovaries decreases – rapidly in some, more slowly in others. A certain proportion of women experience various symptoms during this time, including hot flushes, menstrual irregularity, irritability or anxiety, and sleep disorders. Similar symptoms may be experienced by those who have had surgical removal of their ovaries.

Although the cause of these symptoms is not known to be directly due to estrogen, it has been shown that estrogens can partly relieve these symptoms.

Premarin and other similar estrogen mixture compounds such as Anestrogen, Conestron, Evex, Follestrol, Menotabs, and SK-Estrogens, are primarily prescribed to replace the deficient estrogens. There is some controversy over whether these mixtures or single estrogen compounds such as ethinyl estradiol are more likely to simulate the body's normal estrogens, but at present this has not been resolved.

The most widely publicized, controversy over Premarin and the other estrogens given for menopausal symptoms relates to the possible association with an increased incidence of cancer of the uterus. This has been hotly argued but at the present the information does seem to suggest a somewhat greater risk. The arguments in favor of the use of estrogens include considerations of improved quality of life (i.e. decreased menopausal symptoms) and prevention of fractures (which occur due to bone degeneration or osteoporosis in a certain proportion of women after menopause).

At present, the controversy continues, but there is a greater tendency to use Premarin and related drugs more selectively – for treatment of specific symptoms when required, with general withdrawal except when needed to prevent osteoporosis. One of the more distressing symptoms of the menopause involves decreased secretion in the vaginal area, which can result in painful intercourse due to drying of the mucous membranes in the vagina. The isolated problem is often treated locally with Premarin or other estrogen vaginal cream.

adult dosage The dose varies considerably according to use. For menopausal symptoms, 0.3 to 1.25 mg per day is usually given on a cyclic basis, with 20-23 days on and 7-10 days off the drug each month. The vaginal cream is applied nightly or several times per week.

adverse effects A variety of side effects may occur including nausea or upper gastrointestinal distress, vaginal bleeding or spotting, breast enlargement, weight changes, edema or swelling, headaches and mood changes.

precautions The benefits, indications and risks of the use of this and related drugs should be discussed thoroughly with the prescribing physician. Persons with a history of thrombophlebitis or blood clots in the legs or lungs, or previous breast or uterine cancer or liver disease may be unable to use estrogens.

drug interactions At present, although several theoretical interactions have been suggested, clear cut interactions have not been described.

see essay *Estrogens and Progestogens Used in Hormonal Therapy.*

Principen (brand name for ampicillin). See AMPICILLIN.

Pro-Banthine

generic name

propantheline bromide (available by generic name)

action and uses A drug used to treat ulcers of the stomach and symptoms of gastrointestinal spasm. Pro-Banthine reduces the movement of the muscles of the stomach and intestines and also helps reduce the secretion of acid in the stomach. It is often used in combination with other drugs, particularly antacids, to treat ulcers. It is sometimes used in the treatment of urinary dysfunction.

adult dosage Usually 15 mg just before meals and two 15 mg tablets at bedtime. Pro-Banthine is available in 7.5 mg and 15 mg tablets.

adverse effects Pro-Banthine reduces the secretion of acid in the stomach, but also affects the secretions elsewhere, as in the salivary glands and bronchial tubes. Consequently it may cause dryness of the mouth and drying of bronchial secretions. Other side effects include blurred vision, drowsiness, and difficulty in urinating.

precautions Should be used with caution in individuals with prostate trouble, hiatus hernia, glaucoma, and chronic lung disease.

drug interactions When used with antacids, Pro-Banthine may cause constipation, and its side effects are additive to the similar side effects of antihistamines, cough/cold medicines, and tricyclic antidepressants.

see essay *Drugs for Nausea, Stomach Upset and Ulcers.*

Procainamide (generic name). See PRONESTYL.

Proloid

generic name

thyroglobulin (available by generic name)

action and uses A purified extract of animal thyroid used to replace thyroid hormone in people with a deficiency of thyroid hormone. Thyroid hormones help to regulate many of the body's functions, especially the metabolism, including the rate at which cells use oxygen. In certain diseases of the thyroid such as myxedema (hypothyroidism) and simple goiter, the hormone levels may be reduced and purified hormones from animals, such as Proloid, are used as replacement therapy. In most cases today, the pure hormones, as in Synthroid, are preferred over the gland extracts. Proloid, like other thyroid preparations, has no place in weight control therapy.

adult dosage The dosage must be adjusted to the individual's requirements. Proloid is produced in seven different strengths: 16 mg, 32 mg, 65 mg, 100 mg, 130 mg, 200 mg, and 325 mg. Laboratory tests are usually necessary to determine the correct dosage.

adverse effects If too high a dose of Proloid is given, symptoms of overdose will occur. These include nervousness, sweating, irregular and rapid heartbeat, chest pains (angina) and irregular menstruation.

precautions The required dose of Proloid may vary, so regular checks of thyroid function may be needed. Careful regulation of the dose is also important if high blood pressure or heart disease is also present.

drug interactions When taken with thyroid drugs, certain tricyclic antidepressant drugs such as Elavil and decongestants or drugs for asthma can increase the likelihood of palpitations, rapid heart rate and elevation of the blood pressure.

see essay *Drugs for Thyroid Disorders.*

Promethazine (generic name). See PHENERGAN.

Pronestyl

generic name

procainamide (available by generic name)

action and uses
A drug used to regulate abnormal heart rhythm, and secondarily to increase the heart's efficiency. Pronestyl can decrease the number of extra heart beats, and is sometimes also able to convert an irregular heart rhythm to a regular one and maintain it. It is usually administered orally, except in emergencies, when it may be injected.

adult dosage
Usually highly individualized according to body weight, the specific type of abnormal heart rhythm, and the patient's response to therapy. Per day, the suggested dosage is in the range of 50 mg per kilogram of body weight, given in divided doses at 3-4 hour intervals (usually 300-400 mg every 3-4 hours).

adverse effects
Large doses may cause loss of appetite, nausea, vomiting, diarrhea, mental confusion or hallucinations. These effects can sometimes be prevented by measuring blood levels of the drug. Use may result in a disorder called lupus erythematosus which causes chills and fever, pains in the joints, chest or abdomen, facial rash, and requires discontinuation of the drug. Any of these symptoms should be reported to the doctor promptly.

precautions
People allergic to Novocain (procaine), the local anesthetic frequently used by dentists, are often allergic to this drug. Pronestyl should be monitored carefully in patients with impaired kidney function, and myasthenia gravis.

drug interactions
Pronestyl can be additive to the blood pressure-lowering effects of antihypertensive drugs. The diuretic Diamox, used for glaucoma, can increase the amount of Pronestyl in the blood and the dose may have to be decreased.

see essay
Drugs for Abnormal Heart Rhythm.

Propantheline (generic name). See PRO-BANTHINE.

Propoxyphene (generic name). See DARVON.

Provera

generic name

medroxyprogesterone acetate

action and uses
A female hormone used to treat irregular menstrual cycles and so called "functional" uterine bleeding. It is also used to relieve painful menstruation and occasionally to relieve the tension which frequently occurs before menstruation (pre-menstrual tension). Provera is a synthetic version of the hormone which is normally produced by the female ovary and by the placenta during pregnancy. This or the related progesterone drugs are also used in certain types of severe chronic lung therapy.

adult dosage
The dose varies according to the condition it is used to treat. Usually 5-10 mg per day for 5 to 10 days beginning between the 16th to the 21st days of the menstrual cycle. Provera should never be taken without the advice and supervision of a physician.

adverse effects
The progesterone hormones are believed to have fewer serious side effects than the estrogens. They can cause various menstrual abnormalities, fluid retention, weight changes, skin changes and depression. Liver damage has rarely occurred.

precautions
Provera should not be used by pregnant, potentially pregnant or nursing women, and should not be taken by individuals who have serious liver disease or have had (or have) cancer of the breast, cervix, uterus or ovary. It should be taken with caution by those who have had blood clots in the legs or elsewhere.

drug interactions
Since progestogens such as Provera are seldom used alone or for long periods, drug interactions have not been identified as yet.

see essay
Estrogens and Progestogens used in Hormone Therapy.

Pseudoephedrine (generic name). See SUDAFED.

Pyridium

generic name

phenazopyridine hydrochloride (available by generic name)

action and uses
A drug used to relieve bladder pain caused by infection, injury or surgery of the bladder. It acts to anesthetize the bladder. Although at one time it was thought that Pyridium killed the bacteria which caused bladder infections, it is now known that it only relieves pain. When taken by mouth it is absorbed into the blood and goes through the kidneys and into the bladder where it has its effect. It is then excreted in the urine.

adult dosage
Usually 200 mg, three times per day after meals, only

when bladder pain is present.

adverse effects   The most outstanding effect of Pyridium is that it turns the urine a reddish-orange color, which may stain the underwear. This is perfectly normal and the urine returns to normal when the drug is stopped. In patients with kidney disease the drug may collect in the blood and give a yellowish tinge to the eyes and skin. Pyridium can occasionally upset the stomach, or cause allergic reactions.

precautions   Pyridium should not be taken by patients with severe kidney disease. Pregnant or potentially pregnant or nursing women should ask the physician's advice.

drug interactions   Pyridium can interfere with many urine and blood tests. These should not be done while the drug is being taken.

see essay   *Drugs to Treat Infections.*

Quibron

generic ingredients

bronchodilator = theophylline
expectorant = glyceryl guaiacolate

action and uses   A combination drug used for the treatment of asthma. It contains the bronchodilator theophylline in combination with the expectorant glyceryl guaiacolate. Theophylline is one of the most effective and useful bronchodilator drugs available, if taken in appropriate doses. It is often prescribed generically by itself and is generally less expensive in this form. The expectorant's usefulness in this preparation is not known, since although theoretically it would be useful to liquefy and mobilize secretions in the asthmatic, tests for demonstration of this effect have not been conclusive.

adult dosage   One to two capsules every 6-8 hours. Since the amount of theophylline needed to produce a bronchodilator effect varies considerable from person to person, the dose is usually adjusted according to clinical relief of symptoms, testing of lung function and/or blood levels of the drug theophylline.

adverse effects   If theophylline levels become high, nausea or stomach upset may occur. Less commonly, headaches, palpitations, muscle cramps or jitteriness can be seen, but almost all of these will disappear with lower doses.

precautions   Quibron may be additive to certain over-the-counter drugs used to treat asthma, as well as other drugs given for asthma, so that the treating physician should be aware of all drugs being used.

drug interactions   Both components may affect the clotting system and interact with blood thinning drugs such as Coumadin or heparin. As noted above, Quibron can be additive to other drugs used for treatment of asthma.

see essay   *Drugs for Asthma and Lung Disease.*

Quinidine Sulfate

trade names

> Quinidex, Quinora

action and uses   A drug commonly used to control abnormal or irregular heart rhythms which result in ineffective pumping of the heart and inadequate circulation of blood. The major use of quinidine sulfate, which comes from cinchona bark, is to suppress abnormal and irregular heart rhythms. It is a dangerous drug which should be used only under strict medical supervision. It may eventually be replaced by other drugs since it is not always effective, and it is relatively costly since it must be obtained from tropical countries.

adult dosage   Usually 100-400 mg every two to three hours with careful monitoring. After a normal heart rhythm is restored the usual dosage is 100-200 mg, three to four times per day. It is given by mouth or, rarely, by injection.

adverse effects   Side effects to this drug are unpredictable and they appear in some individuals but not in others. They may include dizziness, nausea, vomiting, diarrhea and breathing problems. Some common allergies can occur. If this occurs a person will also be sensitive to quinine. Taken in excess amounts it may accumulate in the body and cause a condition known as cinchonism. This may result in disturbances in hearing, such as ringing in the ears, changes in vision, stomach upset, skin rashes, local swelling, headache, fever and confusion.

precautions   Quinidine should be used with caution in persons with a history of heart block, and should be avoided by pregnant or potentially pregnant women.

drug interactions   When sodium bicarbonate or certain antacids are used on a regular basis, the dose of quinidine required may be lower; the drug Diamox has the same effect. Quinidine may add to the effects of the anticlotting drug Coumadin and increase the risk of bleeding.

see essay   *Drugs for Abnormal Heart Rhythm.*

Regroton

generic
ingredients

> antihypertensive = reserpine
> diuretic = chlorthalidone

action and uses
A fixed combination drug used to treat high blood pressure. Regroton incoporates two different drugs each of which has an effect on lowering blood pressure. Reserpine acts on the nervous system, to block nerves causing constriction of blood vessels, and chlorthalidone causes loss of salt and water and also dilates the blood vessels. The actions of the drugs together are additive. Although this combination allows the usage of smaller doses of each drug to avoid the possibility of adverse side effects which occur with higher doses, it does not allow for individualization of therapy or identification of the cause of side effects if they occur.

adult dosage
Usually one tablet daily.

adverse effects
Regroton can cause adverse effects related to either of its components. Reserpine can cause depression, nasal stuffiness, stomach upset, and a drop in blood pressure on changing posture (for example, standing up too quickly). The chlorthalidone can cause excessive loss of potassium, especially when taken daily. If this occurs potassium can be replaced either in the diet (extra orange juice, tomato juice, or bananas), or with liquid potassium chloride (KCl). Hygroton also tends to cause an increased blood sugar in those predisposed to diabetes and may increase uric acid levels (the substance in the blood which can cause gout). If used to excess, the diuretic can cause dehydration and may effect kidney function and the amount of waste products in the blood. Allergic rashes may also occur due to chlorthalidone.

precautions
Regroton should be used with caution by patients with gout, diabetes, depression or peptic ulcers. It should be avoided if possible by pregnant or potentially pregnant women. Women taking this drug for long periods should have regular breast examinations.

drug interactions
Drugs for weight loss, asthma, colds, depression and heart conditions may counteract the effect of Regroton to increase the blood pressure and they should be taken together only under the supervision of the physician who prescribed the Regroton. Alcohol and other sedative drugs may also have enhanced effects when taken with Regroton. The chlorthalidone in Regroton can cause excess

potassium loss, which can increase sensitivity to toxic effects of digoxin, and also add to the similar effects of steroids, such as prednisone.

see essays

Drugs for High Blood Pressure. Diuretics.

Reserpine

trade names

> Sandril, Serpasil

action and uses

A commonly used antihypertensive drug which blocks the nerves causing constriction of arterial blood vessels. Formerly used in mental patients, its effectiveness in relieving high blood pressure has made it one of the more widely used drugs. More often, it is given in various combinations such as Ser-Ap-Es, Regroton, or Diupres. Because of a controversial finding of possible association between its use and breast cancer, plus the availability of new drugs such as Inderal, its use has declined. However, since it must be taken only once daily, this fact has tended to maintain it as a popular preparation.

adult dosage

0.125–0.25 mg daily.

adverse effects

A significant number of people do experience side effects, some dose-related. A stuffy nose, gastric upset (or even ulcer) and other gastrointestinal symptoms may occur. Especially in those persons with a history of it, depression or unusual feelings or dreams can be a problem. Sexual function may be altered.

precautions

This drug should be used with caution in persons with a history of peptic ulcer, severe allergic sinusitis or depression. Women taking this drug for long periods should have regular breast examinations.

drug interactions

The decongestants in nasal sprays, cough/cold medicines and drugs for asthma can counteract the blood pressure lowering effect. The sedating effects, if present, can be additive to tranquilizers and alcohol.

see essay

Drugs for High Blood Pressure.

Ritalin

generic name

> methylphenidate

action and uses

A stimulant drug which is, at present, most commonly used in the treatment of hyperkinetic children, and although effective, is quite controversial. It is also used on occasion in the treatment of mild depression although its effectiveness for this has not been clearly established. It has also been used, uncommonly, as a drug to help decrease appetite and promote weight loss. It is quite similar in its effects to the amphetamine drugs, and since it has been substituted for them by drug abusers, it requires special prescriptions similar to those for narcotic drugs.

adult dosage 10 mg once to three times daily. Dosage in children differs and varies. Other sources should be consulted.

adverse effects Nervousness, decreased appetite and difficulty sleeping are the most common side effects, although dizziness, palpitations, increased blood pressure, headache, and stomach upset may also occur. Prolonged use can cause weight loss and habituation, so that discontinuing the drug can cause withdrawal symptoms such as depression.

precautions This drug should not be used by persons with anxiety or nervousness, high blood pressure or any type of heart disease, epilepsy, or problems with drug or alcohol abuse.

drug dependence Prolonged use may result in dependence on Ritalin.

drug interactions Ritalin can counteract the effects of antihypertensive drugs. It can be additive to increase the likelihood of side effects when used with decongestants and nasal sprays. It also counteracts the effect of anticonvulsant drugs such as Dilantin.

see essay *Antidepressants and Lithium.*

Robaxin-750

generic name

methocarbamol

action and uses A muscle relaxant which acts on the central nervous system and is similar to minor tranquilizers such as meprobamate. Robaxin is used in the relief of low back pain and other pains of muscles and joints. The way Robaxin acts to relax muscles and relieve pain is not known, although it is known that it does not act directly on the muscles.

adult dosage Usually 1-2 grams four times a day, for the first 3 days, followed by 1-2 grams 3 times a day.

adverse effects Robaxin may cause lightheadedness, dizziness, drowsiness, nausea, blurred vision, headache and fever. Some people may develop allergic reactions including skin rash, itching and hives.

precautions Robaxin should not be used in pregnant, potentially pregnant or nursing women. It may infere with driving or operating machinery.

drug interactions
The sedative effects can be additive to the effects of tranquilizers, sleeping pills and alcohol.

see essay
Non-Narcotic Pain Relievers.

Robitet

generic name

tetracycline (available by generic name)

action and uses

One of the most commonly used oral antibiotics. In the generic form it was the 4th most frequently prescribed drug in 1976. There are a number of tetracycline drugs available, but most are comparable in their actions and side effects except for Minocin and Vibramycin. Robitet (tetracycline) is known as a "broad spectrum" antibiotic because it can be used in a wide variety of different infections, although it is the first choice drug in a very few common infections. It acts by stopping the production of proteins in sensitive bacterial cells with little effect on human cells. Tetracycline is currently very commonly used in low doses to inhibit the bacteria on the face which are believed to contribute to acne. It is also frequently used by those with chronic bronchitis or other lung disease. Less frequently it is used to treat urinary tract infections or venereal disease when penicillin allergy is present. It has no effect on viral illnesses, including colds, or fungus infections.

adult dosage

The usual oral dose is 250 or 500 mg every six hours for a prescribed number of days as specified by the physician. It is very important to take this on an empty stomach. The dose may vary in some cases such as acne, where it may be lower.

adverse effects

Tetracycline commonly can cause various gastrointestinal symptoms including nausea and vomiting, burning stomach or belching, cramps and diarrhea. The latter symptom is often due to the fact that tetracycline inhibits some bacteria in the lower intestine and elsewhere and allows overgrowth of other bacteria (normally held in check) and minor fungi. This can also result in vaginal infections, anorectal itching and a sore mouth (thrush). These symptoms tend to disappear when the drug is discontinued. Less commonly, tetracycline can cause rashes, or other allergic reactions and sensitivity of the skin to sunlight, causing rashes (photosensitivity). It can also tend to worsen certain types of kidney disease, and rarely cause liver damage or blood cell abnormalities.

precautions

Tetracycline should not be taken by pregnant or potentially pregnant or nursing women, and should be used with caution when significant liver or kidney disease is present. This antibiotic, like all others, should be taken for the time period directed, and every dose should be taken. Failure to do this can result in inadequate treatment of the infection, recurrence or development of resistant infections.

drug interactions

The most common drug interaction is between tetracycline and antacids or milk products, since the tetracycline binds to these and does not get into the body. Tetracycline can potentially increase the effect of the anticoagulant Coumadin and increase the hazard of bleeding.

see essay

Drugs to Treat Infections.

Salutensin

generic
ingredients

diuretic = hydroflumethiazide
antihypertensive = reserpine

action and uses

Salutensin is a combination product used to treat mild to moderate high blood pressure. It combines a thiazide-type diuretic, hydroflumethiazide, which causes a dilation of blood vessels and loss of excess salt and water, with reserpine, a drug which helps block the sympathetic or adrenalin-like causes of high blood pressure. Hydroflumethiazide is like many other thiazide diuretics such as hydrochlorothiazide, Esidrix or Diuril. Ideally, this combination is started only after it is determined that both ingredients are really needed to control blood pressure.

adult dosage

One tablet daily or twice daily.

adverse effects

Side effects may develop due to either drug which makes use of this combination more problematic. The hydroflumethiazide can cause excess potassium loss in some, resulting in weakness, lethargy or dizziness. It can also elevate the blood sugar in those predisposed to diabetes, and elevate the serum uric acid and predispose to gout. In some, reserpine can cause depression or anxiety, peptic ulcer and nasal stuffiness, and occasionally dizziness associated with rapid postural changes.

precautions

Use of this drug in persons with a history of depression or peptic ulcer should involve careful medical supervision. Many cough/cold medicines or nasal sprays should be avoided. It should be avoided if possible by pregnant or potentially pregnant women. Women taking this drug for long periods should have regular breast examinations.

drug interactions The potassium loss caused by the diuretic may increase the likelihood of toxicity to digoxin if the two drugs are used together. Further, the diuretic component causes high calcium retention, so calcium supplements, vitamin D and antacids containing calcium can cause elevated calcium in the blood. Use of many anti-allergy, asthma or cough/cold medicines or nasal sprays containing phenylephrine, ephedrine or phenylpropanolamine may raise the blood pressure and counteract the effect of this drug. The blood pressure lowering effect of Salutensin can be additive to other antihypertensive drugs (such as Inderal) as well as to general anesthetics, and can cause excessively low blood pressure.

see essays *Drugs for High Blood Pressure. Diuretics.*

Septra

generic ingredients

> antibacterials = sulfamethoxazole, trimethoprim

action and uses A fixed combination drug used to treat infections of the urinary tract. It is the same drug as Bactrim, another trade name. Septra combines a sulfa drug, which is particularly effective against the bacteria which commonly affect the bladder and kidney, with a chemical antibacterial drug which acts against the same bacteria. Together the two drugs are more effective than either one alone, since each inhibits a separate enzyme in the bacteria, which decreases the likelihood of resistance developing. This combination is also finding use in certain other common diseases, such as typhoid fever.

adult dosage Usually one double strength tablet, or two ordinary tablets, or four teaspoonfuls of liquid, every 12 hours, for 10 to 14 days. It may be used for longer periods in chronic urinary tract infections.

adverse effects This drug may sometimes cause nausea, vomiting or other gastrointestinal symptoms as well as headaches or dizziness. Like all sulfa drugs, Septra may cause allergic reactions such as rashes, as well as very serious, life-threatening reactions with fever, severe rash, and kidney failure. Abnormalities of the blood cells may also occur.

precautions It is always important to drink plenty of water while taking this drug to prevent crystal formation in the kidney. If any fever, nausea or rash occur after starting the drug, it should be discontinued and the doctor notified. It should be avoided in persons with sever kidney disease and G6PD deficiency (a red blood cell disease). As in the treatment of all infections, it is important to take the drug for the full time recommended to prevent recurrence of the infection.

drug interactions   As with many sulfa drugs, Septra may increase the effect of oral antidiabetic drugs (to cause low blood sugar), and Dilantin, Butazolidin, and phenobarbital to increase the likelihood of toxicity to these drugs.

see essay   *Drugs to Treat Infections.*

Ser-Ap-Es

generic
ingredients

> antihypertensive = reserpine
> diuretic = hydrochlorothiazide
> vasodilator = hydralazine

action and uses   A fixed combination drug used to treat high blood pressure. Ser-Ap-Es incorporates three different drugs each of which has an effect on lowering blood pressure. Reserpine acts on the nervous system to block nerves causing constriction of blood vessels, hydrochlorothiazide causes loss of salt and water and also dilates the blood vessels, and hydralazine dilates the blood vessels. The actions of the drugs together are additive. Although this combination allows the usage of smaller doses of each drug to avoid the possibility of adverse side effects which occur with higher doses, it does not allow for individualization of therapy or identification of the cause of side effects if they occur.

adult dosage   It is seldom that a multiple of the dosage of all three components of Ser-Ap-Es in fact approximates the best dose of each drug for controlling blood pressure and minimizing side effects. The usual dosage is 1-2 tablets twice a day but this must be carefully determined for each individual patient.

adverse effects   Ser-Ap-Es can cause side effects related to any of its three components. Reserpine can cause depression, nasal stuffiness, stomach upset, and a drop in blood pressure on changing posture (for example, standing up too quickly). The side effects of hydrochlorothiazide are not usually prominent due to the relatively low dose; and the side effects due to hydralazine are usually not present due to the reserpine component, although allergic rashes may occur to either.

precautions Ser-Ap-Es should be used with caution by patients with gout or diabetes, depression or peptic ulcers. It should be avoided if possible by pregnant or potentially pregnant women. Women taking this drug for long periods should have regular breast examinations.

drug interactions Drugs for weight loss, asthma, colds, depression and heart conditions may interact with Ser-Ap-Es to increase the blood pressure and they should be taken together only under the supervision of the physician who prescribed the Ser-Ap-Es. Alcohol and other sedative drugs may also have enhanced effects when taken with Ser-Ap-Es. The thiazide diuretic may increase loss of potassium, which is additive to the effects of steroids such as prednisone, and which also can increase sensitivity to the toxic effects of digoxin.

see essays *Drugs for High Blood Pressure. Diuretics.*

Serax

generic name

oxazepam

action and uses A minor tranquilizer used in the treatment of mild to severe anxiety, and sometimes to relieve the symptoms of alcohol withdrawal. Chemically similar to the tranquilizers Valium, Librium and Tranxene, Serax may, in some cases, be preferable because it does not share their tendency to accumulate in the body.

adult dosage The usual dose of Serax ranges from 10-15 mg 2 to 4 times per day, to 15-30 mg 3 to 4 times per day. For those who experience anxiety only intermittently, one dose may be sufficient.

adverse effects On the whole, Serax is a fairly safe tranquilizer. Its side effects may include sleepiness, lethargy, dizziness, fatigue, depression, irritability, headache or nausea. These effects can sometimes be eliminated by lowering the dose. Other side effects, such as allergic skin reactions, are unusual.

precautions Because of the possible connection between similar drugs and birth defects, the package insert for Serax warns against its use by pregnant or potentially pregnant women. It may interfere with driving or operating machinery.

drug dependence Psychological and/or physical dependence are possible with extended use of this drug.

drug interactions

The sedative effects of Serax can be increased by alcohol, sleeping pills, other tranquilizers, antidepressants, and antihistamines.

see essay

Minor Tranquilizers.

Sinequan

generic name

doxepin

action and uses

A commonly prescribed antidepressent drug. Like Elavil and Tofranil, it belongs to a group of closely-related drugs called tricyclic antidepressents, and is used to treat certain types of moderately severe and long-standing depression. The tricyclic antidepressents are not true tranquilizers, although they can cause some sedation. The antidepressant effect of Sinequan may take days or weeks to appear, although no temporary sedative and other side effects occur immediately.

adult dosage

The effective dose of Sinequan is highly individualized and dosage adjustment may take one or two months. Initially the dose is usually 25-75 mg per day, and may be increased to 150 mg per day. (The dose may be lower for elderly patients.) Because the drug is long-acting and may cause some sedation, it is usually taken just once a day, at bedtime.

adverse effects

Initially, Sinequan may cause dry mouth, blurred vision, drowsiness, constipation and difficulty in urination. These effects are especially a problem in older people, but they tend to disappear in 3-4 weeks. Other significant side effects may include effects on the heart rhythm, and sometimes confusion or dizziness.

precautions

Sinequan should be taken with caution by persons with glaucoma, prostate gland problems, liver or heart disease, epilepsy or hyperthyroid condition. It should not be taken by pregnant or potentially pregnant or nursing women. The drowsiness may interfere with driving or operating machinery.

drug interactions

Sinequan can cause oversedation when taken in combination with alcohol, sleeping pills, tranquilisers, antihistamines and drugs containing narcotics. It can add to the side effects of antispasmodic drugs and decrease the effects of drugs to lower blood pressure such as Ismelin. It can dangerously interfere with drugs to regulate heart rhythm, thyroid drugs and drugs of the MAO inhibitor family (such as Marplan, Parnate and Nardil). Taken with drugs of the latter type, or with the sedative Placidyl, Sinequan can cause delirium.

see essay

Antidepressants and Lithium.

Singlet

generic
ingredients

decongestant = phenylephrine hydrochloride
antihistamine = chlorpheniramine
 pain reliever = acetaminophen

action and uses

A combination drug used to treat symptoms of colds and allergies. The antihistamine and decongestant help relieve nasal congestion and stop runny nose. The acetaminophen can both decrease fever and act as a mild pain reliever.

adult dosage

The usual dose is one tablet 3 to 4 times per day.

adverse effects

Side effects may include drowsiness due to the antihistamine and possibly palpitation due to the decongestants.

precautions

Singlet should be avoided by pregnant or potentially pregnant women and nursing mothers. Driving or operating heavy equipment may be hazardous if sedation is an effect of this medication. Persons taking medicine for high blood pressure or heart trouble should check with their physicians before using, since the decongestants may elevate the blood pressure. Repeated use for any period more than 2 to 4 days is not desirable in most cases. Excessive doses of the acetaminophen can cause liver damage.

drug interactions

The sedative effects of the antihistamine, can be additive to any other sedating drugs such as tranquilizers and alcohol. The decongestants can raise the blood pressure and thus counteract the effect of any drug used to treat high blood pressure. Like most of the drugs of this type, Singlet may add to the effects of antispasmodic drugs used for stomach disorders, such as Pro-Bantine and Librax. This can cause excessive mouth dryness and difficulty in urinating.

see essay

Drugs for Coughs and Colds.

Slow-K

generic name

potassium chloride (available by generic name)

action and uses

A special preparation of potassium chloride (KCl) used to replace potassium in cases of potassium loss. Slow-K is usually prescribed for patients who eliminate too much potassium because they are taking a diuretic ("water pill") for high blood pressure or some other reason. The active chemical ingredient, potassium chloride, is contained in a wax matrix to keep it from being released into the system too quickly. This is believed to prevent ulceration of the stomach and intestines which can occur if potassium is released too quickly. Whether this actually works has been questioned. The risk of ulceration, the cost, and the many pills required each day make it doubtful that this form of potassium is better than liquid KCl or powder preparations.

adult dosage The dose varies from person to person and must be determined by the physician. The usual dose is 5 tablets (40 milliequivalents) to 10 tablets a day, which is a disadvantage in taking this preparation.

adverse effects Slow-K can produce severe ulceration of the stomach and intestines if there is any obstruction to its movement through the sytem. Because it is specially designed to be released slowly, however, this is not a common problem. It may also cause nausea, vomiting, intestinal cramps, and diarrhea.

precautions This drug should be used with careful supervision in those persons with severe kidney disease, severe diabetes, and water deprivation.

drug interactions Slow-K should not be used with drugs which retain potassium, such as spironolactone (Aldactone, Aldactezide) or triamterene (Dyazide, Dyrenium).

see essays *Drugs for High Blood Pressure. Diuretics. Vitamins and Minerals.*

Sorbitrate

generic name

isosorbide dinitrate (available by generic name)

action and uses A drug which is used to relieve pain in the treatment of angina pectoris, a heart condition characterized by pain (usually after exercise or emotion) in the chest or arm. The pain is due to lack of oxygen, carried by the blood. Sorbitrate acts in two ways: to open up the (often partly blocked) blood vessels to the heart, and to dilate peripheral blood vessels to decrease the work the heart must do.

Sorbitrate is sometimes also used to treat conditions where blood circulation is poor, such as Raynaud's disease, and in certain other heart failure conditions.

adult dosage For acute attacks the usual dosage is 2.5 to 10mg; the tablets are placed under the tongue and allowed to dissolve. The tablets each contain either 2.5 mg or 5 mg. For regular use tablets containing 5 mg, 10 mg, or 20 mg are *swallowed* to reduce the frequency of anginal attacks. For this purpose the usual dosage is 5-30 mg taken four times per day by swallowing. Long-acting tablets and long-acting capsules, called Tembrids, containing 40 mg isosorbide dinitrate are also available. These should be taken every 6 to 12 hours.

adverse effects

Flushing is very common and is due to increased blood flow to the skin. Throbbing headache often occurs and is also associated with changes in blood flow. A feeling of faintness of dizziness can occur (particularly in hot weather) more commonly in persons with high blood pressure.

precautions

If more than 2 or 3 tablets do not relieve the pain, the doctor should be notified at once.

drug interactions

Excessive alcohol intake tends to dilate blood vessels and increase the action of isosorbide, as do certain antihypertensive drugs, such as Apresoline.

see essays

Drugs used to Prevent of Treat Circulation Problems. Drugs for Angina Pectoris.

Stelazine

generic name

trifluoperazine

action and uses

One of a large family of drugs known as phenothiazines. Stelazine is a major tranquilizer, or "antipsychotic" drug, primarliy used in the treatment of serious physcological disorders. Though not capable of curing the underlying illness, Stelazine and the other drugs in this group do relieve the severe thought disorders (such as disorientation, delusions and hallucinations) that characterize schizophrenia and manic-depressive psychoses, severe alcohol withdrawal, some cases of senility, some neurological diseases, and the effects of certain drugs such as LSD and amphetamines.

adult dosage

For the treatment of thought disorders the initial dose may range from 2 to 15 mg per day, but may eventually go as high as 50+ mg per day in some cases. The dose is likely to be highly individualized, because sensitivity to the drug varies widely from person to person. Generally speaking, however, the dose tends to be lower for older people and, whatever the patient's age, it may usually be taken just once a day and occasionally omitted on weekends.

adverse effects
Stelazine may produce a number of significant side effects and can occasionally cause some serious drug reactions. Its use, therefore, must be carefully supervised. Unlike the other phenothiazine drugs such as Thorazine, Stelazine causes only mild sedation and seldom causes significant fall in the blood pressure. It has a greater tendency, however, to produce tremors and restlessness, so-called Parkinsonian side effects due to their similarity to Parkinson's disease. These effects can usually be decreased by addition of anti-Parkinsonian drugs like Cogentin, Stelazine can cause jaundice, skin rash, or a decrease in the white blood cell count (which increases the patient's vulnerability to infection) and the drug must be discontinued. These side effects and adverse reactions are not common. A serious side effect, called "tardive dyskinesia" which is characterized by uncontrollable movements of the tongue and lips, occasionally occurs when the drug is discontinued.

precautions
Prolonged use of Stelazine requires regular medical evaluation at intervals.

drug interactions
Oversedation is possible when Stelazine is taken in combination with alcohol, other sedatives and tranquilizers, sleeping pills, antidepressants, antihistamines and drugs containing narcotics. Stelazine can counteract the blood pressure-lowering effect of the antihypertensive drugs Ismelin and Aldomet.

see essay
Major Tranquilizers.

Sudafed

generic name

pseudoephedrine (available by generic name)

action and uses
Sudafed is a very popular, commonly prescribed decongestant which is used in the treatment of various allergic conditions such as allergic sinusitis or blocked eustachian tubes (stuffy ears), as well as for relief of similar symptoms associated with a cold. It is occasionally used in treatment of asthmatic symptoms. Prolonged or continued use may result in decreased effectiveness.

adult dosage
30-60 mg orally 3 to 4 times per day.

adverse effects
Occasionally some stimulation, insomnia or jitteriness may be noted, although drowsiness or headache may also occur.

precautions
In the case of people who are taking medication for high

blood pressure or heart trouble, Sudafed should only be used after consultation with a physician. Some people may experience pounding of the heart (palpitations).

drug interactions   Sudafed can interact with drugs used to treat high blood pressure and counteract their effects. It is also similar, and therefore additive to ingredients in nasal sprays and in certain drugs given for asthma; their combined use should usually be confirmed with a physician.

see essay   *Drugs for Coughs and Colds.*

Sulfamethoxazole (generic name). See GANTANOL.

Sulfisoxazole (generic name). See GANTRISIN.

Sumycin (brand name). See TETRACYCLINE.

Synalar cream and ointment

generic name

fluocinolone

action and uses   A commonly used topical preparation of a synthetic corticosteroid, or cortisone-like drug. It is used primarily because of its anti-inflammatory effects in the treatment of many types of skin disorders such as psoriasis, certain types of neurodermatitis and a variety of other conditions where there is no infection. In many cases, the effects are dramatic. Because it retards formation of scar tissue, it can also prevent scarring.

adult dosage   The preparation is applied sparingly 2-3 times daily. It is available in ointments, lotions, and creams in several strengths, depending upon where it is to be used.

adverse effects   If the preparation is not used for long periods or on infected areas, there are virtually no important adverse effects; however, if the preparations are used for long intervals on the face, they can cause eruptions and redness. If Synalar preparations are used for long periods on a large portion of the body, the corticosteroid can be absorbed and get into the body. This can cause weight gain, ulcers or stomach upset, decreased resistance to infection and stress, and can be quite hazardous. If used on an infected area of the skin it can help the infection spread, and it can be very hazardous if used for any viral skin lesions such as herpes (cold sores), shingles or chickenpox.

precautions   Do not use for long periods of time or on large areas of the body except under continued medical supervision. If a skin eruption worsens with continued use, the physician should be notified and the preparation discontinued.

drug interactions No significant interactions will occur although other topical preparations placed on the same skin area may interfere with effects.

see essays *Steroids or Cortisone-like Drugs. Drugs for Skin and Local Disorders.*

Synalgos-DC

generic ingredients

narcotic pain reliever = dihydro codeine
sedative = promethazine
pain relievers = aspirin, phenacetin
mild stimulant = caffeine

action and uses A combination product used to relieve pain. This particular combination contains both narcotic and non-narcotic pain relievers as well as a major tranquilizer which was added as a sedative. A similar product, Synalgos, is identical except for the absence of the narcotic. Whether all of these components act together to give greater relief of pain and anxiety than the less costly codeine or aspirin with codiene is not known. The problematic side effects of some ingredients tends to make such a mixture less desirable than simpler drugs.

adult dosage One or two capsules every 4 to 6 hours as needed for pain.

adverse effects Undesired effects can result from several of the components. The dihydrocodeine can cause constipation and both it and the aspirin can cause stomach upset. The promethazine, though present in small doses can cause sedation with repeated doses, along with the narcotic. Allergies, effects on the white blood count and jaundice can rarely occur, as with other major tranquilizers. Allergies can also occur to either the aspirin, phenacetin or codeine. Prolonged use of this phenacetin-containing drug can also cause kidney damage, and the dihydrocodeine can be habituating.

precautions If sedation occurs, driving or operating heavy machinery may be hazardous. This drug should be avoided in pregnant, potentially pregnant and nursing women, and by those sensitive to aspirin, codeine, or phenothiazines.

drug dependence Synalgos-DC may cause physcological and/or physical dependence so prolonged use should be avoided to prevent habituation.

drug interactions The sedative effects of the dihydrocodeine and promethazine can add to the effects of other tranquilizers, sedatives, alcohol or sleeping pills. Aspirin adds to the effects of oral anticoagulants, increasing risk of bleeding, and to the effects of cortisone-like drugs, increasing the risk of peptic ulcer.

see essay | *Narcotic Pain Relievers.*

Synthroid

generic name

> levothyroxine (available by generic name)

action and uses — A synthetic form of thyroid hormone. Thyroid hormones help to regulate many of the body's functions, especially the metabolism, including the rate at which cells use oxygen. In certain diseases of the thyroid, such as myxedema (hypothyroidism) and simple goiter, the hormone levels may be reduced and synthetic hormones, such as Synthroid, are used as replacement therapy. In most cases today, the pure hormones, such as Synthroid, are preferred over the animal gland extracts. Synthroid, like other thyroid preparations, has no place in weight control therapy.

adult dosage — The dosage must be adjusted to the individual's requirements. Synthroid is produced in six different strengths. Synthroid tablets are ten times stronger than other thyroid preparations and cannot be simply substituted for them. Laboratory tests are usually necessary to determine the correct dosage.

adverse effects — If too high a dose of Synthroid is given, symptoms of overdose will occur. These include nervousness, sweating, irregular and rapid heartbeats, chest pains (angina) and, in women, irregular menstruation.

precautions — The required dose of Synthroid may vary so regular checks of thyroid function may be needed. Careful regulation of the dose is also important if high blood pressure or heart disease is also present.

drug interactions — When taken with thyroid drugs, certain tricyclic antidepressant drugs such as Elavil and decongestants or drugs for asthma can increase the likelihood of palpitations, rapid heart rate and elevation of the blood pressure.

see essay | *Drugs for Thyroid Disorders.*

Talwin

generic name

> pentazocine

action and uses	A pain reliever closely related in some respects to the narcotic analgesics, although it is not yet subject to narcotic restrictions. Like codeine, Talwin is used for relief of moderate pain, but it is more expensive than codeine and appears to offer few advantages. Its potential side effects (see below) and its cost tend to limit its usefulness, although it does offer an alternative strong oral analgesic when such a drug is needed, as it is sometimes in cases of terminal cancer.
adult dosage	Talwin may be given by intramuscular injection, or taken orally in doses of 15-60 mg every 3-6 hours as needed for pain.
adverse effects	Talwin can depress breathing, and, like codeine, can cause constipation, nausea, drowsiness and dizziness. Additionally, unlike most narcotic drugs, Talwin can increase blood pressure and heart work, and also can produce unpleasant sensations of anxiety and/or strange thoughts and hallucinations. Allergic skin rashes are another possible side effect.
precautions	Talwin should be avoided by patients with severe respiratory disorders, a history of mental disorders, or epilepsy, or in pregnant, potentially pregnant, or nursing women.
drug dependence	Talwin can cause psychological and/or physical dependence.
drug interactions	Talwin may incrase the sedative effect of tranquilizers, sleeping pills, antidepressants and sedatives, and alcohol.
see essay	*Non-Narcotic Pain Relievers.*

Tandearil

generic name	oxyphenbutazone
action and uses	A drug used to reduce inflammation, especially in the joints. Tandearil relieves the painful symptoms of inflammation but does not cure the disease which causes the inflammation. It is not known how it works. It is not a steroid hormone and is not related to steroids, although its anti-inflammatory actions are similar. Because of very serious side effects it is used only when milder drugs, such as aspirin, do not relieve the symptoms of inflamation. It is useful in treating isolated severe joint pains of inflammed tendons and joints, occasionally for acute gout, and for acute flare-ups of rheumatoid arthritis.
adult dosage	The dosage of Tandearil varies from person to person and

must be determined by the physician for each individual case. It is available in 100 mg tablets, and the daily dose ranges from 300-600 mg, usually taken in divided doses with meals or milk.

While Tandearil is an effective and useful drug it is also a dangerous and poisonous drug. Many severe reactions occur, particularly if it used for longer than 7 days, especially in persons over the age of 60. It may poison the bone marrow and prevent the body from producing both red and white blood cells, thereby causing anemia and loss of resistance to infection. If such a reaction occurs the effects may be irreversible if the drug is not stopped immediately. Hives, skin rashes, itching and sores in and around the mouth can be signs of serious reactions to the drug and should be reported to the physician immediately. Tandearil also may cause stomach upsets, nausea, vomiting and indigestion, though this may be avoided by taking it with meals. It can also cause liver damage and fluid retention.

precautions

Tanderail should not be used by children under age 14, pregnant, potentially pregnant or nursing women. It should never be used for more then 7 days in any person over the age of 60 unless specifically ordered by, and discussed with, a physician, and should be followed with regular blood counts. It should be used cautiously in persons who have stomach or intestinal trouble or ulcers.

drug interactions

Tanderail interacts with many drugs, including antidiabetic drugs, other anti-inflammatory drugs such as Motrin, sulfa drugs, Dilantin and Coumadin, increasing the risk of toxicity of each.

see essay

Drugs for Pain with Inflammation.

Tedral

generic
ingredients

bronchodilators = theophylline,
ephedrine
sedative = phenobarbital

action and uses

A combination of two drugs which relax the bronchi plus phenobarbital used to treat asthma. Theophylline and ephedrine both act on the muscles of the bronchi, relax them, and open up the airways. Phenobarbital theoretically provides a mild sedative for anxious asthmatic patients and counteracts any stimulant effect of the ephedrine. However, neither effect is proven or even likely at the small dose of phenobarbital used. Most often, theophylline alone in proper doses is equally effective, less costly, and has fewer side effects. Further, this fixed combination does not allow dose adjustment.

adult dosage 1 or 2 tablets every four hours (to treat attacks or to prevent them).

adverse effects Adverse effects from the ephedrine component can include nervousness, high blood pressure, fast heart rate, or palpitations. The theophylline can cause nausea, headaches or muscle cramps, and also palpitations. The phenobarbital can cause allergic reactions.

precautions Tedral should be used cautiously in people who have heart disease or high blood pressure. It can be additive to certain over-the-counter drugs for asthma so the prescribing physician should be aware of all drugs being used, including aerosols or inhalers.

drug interactions The ephedrine can be additive (and thus increase side effects) to drugs for coughs and colds, but can counteract antihypertensive drugs.

The theophylline and phenobarbital can interact with anticoagulant drugs like Coumadin to decrease their effect.

see essay *Drugs for Asthma and Lung Disease.*

Teldrin

generic name

chlorpheniramine (available by generic name)

action and uses A commonly prescribed antihistamine which is frequently used to treat allergic conditions, especially allergic rhinitis, sinusitis or conjunctivitis (redness of the eye). It shares the effects of most other antihistamines by blocking the effects of histamines and thus can decrease itching of the skin due to allergies, hives or rashes. It also can sometimes have a sedating effect, although it is not customarily used for this. It is not useful for treatment of asthma. It is usually much less expensive in generic form, as chlorpheniramine.

adult dosage Teldrin is available in long-acting 12 mg capsules. The usual oral dose is one 12 mg capsule once or twice daily as needed for treatment of allergic conditions.

adverse effects Although possibly less frequently than with some other antihistamines, Teldrin may also cause significant sedation in some people. Other side effects are relatively rare, but can include dry mouth, blurred vision, or difficulty in urinating, especially in older persons or those with glaucoma or prostate trouble.

drug interactions Teldrin is additive to other sedative or tranquilizing drugs and alcohol. It is also additive to other antispasmodic drugs used to treat ulcers or stomach problems, such as Pro-Banthine or Librax, to cause excessive dry mouth, constipation and difficulty in urinating.

precautions The sedative effects may interfere with driving or operating machinery. This drug should be used with caution in those with glaucoma or prostate trouble. It should also be avoided by pregnant or potentially pregnant women and nursing mothers.

see essay *Antihistamines.*

Tenuate

generic name

diethylpropion (available by generic name)

action and uses An appetite suppressant used as an aid in weight reduction. Its effect in decreasing the appetite tends to diminish after 7-14 days. Its true effectiveness in causing weight loss can be questioned. Like amphetamine sulfate, to which it is related, it also stimulates the nervous system, producing an increase in energy and mental alertness and a lift in mood. Though Tenuate is less effective in suppressing appetite than amphetamine sulfate, it is probably preferable because it may have less tendency to cause dependence.

adult dosage Usually 25 mg before meals, 3 times daily.

adverse effects Like amphetamine sulfate, Tenuate can cause dry mouth, nervousness, headache, anxiety, nausea, vomiting, rapid, irregular heart beat and elevation of the blood pressure. (In most patients, however, the side effects of Tenuate on the nervous system and cardiovascular system are less marked than they are with amphetamine sulfate). Withdrawal symptoms of fatigue and depression are likely when the drug is stoppped, particularly if it has been taken in doses exceeding those prescribed.

precautions Tenuate should only be used for short periods under careful supervision. It should not be used by anyone with any type of heart disease or irregular heart rhythm or high blood pressure.

drug dependence As with amphetamine sulfate, Tenuate can cause severe psychological and/or physical dependence, and tolerance to its effects develops quickly.

drug interactions Tenuate can counteract the effect of drugs for high blood pressure, and some drugs used to regulate heart rhythms.

271

It can be additive and increase the likelihood of side effects when used with decongestants or nasal sprays and drugs for asthma.

see essay   *Stimulants and Drugs for Weight Loss.*

Terothyroxine (generic name). See SYNTHROID.

Tetracycline

trade names

Achromycin-V, Retet, Robitet, Sumycin, Panmycin, Tetrex.

action and uses   One of the most commonly used oral antibiotics. In the generic form it was the 4th most frequently prescribed drug in 1976. There are a number of tetracycline drugs available, but most are comparable in their actions and side effects except for Minocin and Vibramycin. Tetracyline is known as a "broad spectrum" antibiotic because it can be used in a wide variety of different infections, although it is the first choice drug in very few common infections. It acts by stopping the production of proteins in sensitive bacterial cells with little effect on human cells. Tetracycline is currently very commonly used in low doses to inhibit the bacteria on the face which are believed to contribute to acne. It is also frequently used by those with chronic bronchitis or other lung disease. Less frequently it is used to treat urinary tract infections or venereal disease when penicillin allergy is present. It has no effect on viral illnesses, including colds, or fungus infections.

adult dosage   The usual oral dose in 250 or 500 mg every six hours for a prescribed number of days as specified by the physician. It is very important to take this on an empty stomach. The dose may vary in some cases such as acne, where it may be lower.

adverse effects   Tetracycline commonly can cause various gastrointestinal symptoms including nausea and vomiting, burning stomach or belching, cramps and diarrhea. The latter symptom is often due to the fact that tetracycline inhibits some bacteria in the lower intestine and elsewhere, and thus allows overgrowth of other bacteria (normally held in check) and minor fungi. This can also result in vaginal infections, anorectal itching and a sore mouth (thrush). These symptoms tend to disappear when the drug is discontinued. Less commonly, tetracycline can cause rashes, or other allergic reactions and sensitivity of the skin to sunlight, causing rashes (photosensitivity). It can also tend to worsen certain types of kidney disease, and rarely cause liver damage or blood cell abnormalities.

precautions   Tetracycline should not be taken by pregnant or potentially pregnant or nursing women, and should be used with caution when significant liver or kidney disease is present. This antibiotic, like all others, should be taken for the time period directed, and every dose should be taken. Failure to do this can result in inadequate treatment of the infection, recurrence or development of resistant infections.

drug interactions   The most common drug interaction is between tetracycline and antacids or milk products, since the tetracycline binds to these and does not get into the body. Tetracycline can potentially increase the effect of the anticoagulant Coumadin and increase the hazard of bleeding.

see essay   *Drugs to treat Infections.*

Theophylline (generic name). See ELIXOPHYLLIN.

Thorazine

generic name

chlorpromazine (available by generic name)

action and uses   The prototype of a large family of major tranquilizers, or "anti-psychotic" drugs, primarily used in the treatment of serious psychological disorders. Though not capable of curing the underlying illness, thorazine and the other drugs in this group do relieve the severe thought disorders (such as disorientation, delusions, and hallucinations) that characterize schizophrenia and manic-depressive psychoses, severe alcohol withdrawal, some cases of senility, some neurological disease, and the effects of certain drugs such as LSD and amphetamine. First introduced as a "tranquilizer" in the early 1950s, Thorazine revolutionized the treatment of mental patients by making it possible for them to receive therapy in the community rather than being confined to locked hospital wards.

    Thorazine also has sedative effects, but is usually used for this purpose only when the patient is also suffering from a thought disorder. Thorazine can also be used to decrease nausea and vomiting, and to stop hiccoughs (when they cannot be stopped in other ways).

adult dosage   For the treatment of thought disorders, the initial dose of Thorazine may be 50-200 mg per day, eventually rising to 750-1000 mg per day in some cases. The dose is likely to be highly individualized, because sensitivity to the drug varies widely from person to person. Generally speaking, how-

273

ever, the dose tends to be lower for older people, and, whatever the patient's age, it may usually be taken just once a day (often at bedtime, to take advantage of its sedative effect) when used over a long period of time.

adverse effects Thorazine may produce a number of significant side effects, and can occasionally cause serious drug reactions. Its use, therefore, must be carefully supervised. When first taken, Thorazine is likely to produce heavy sedation, a sensation of mental dullness, and, in some cases, blurred vision, dry mouth and constipation. These effects usually diminish if the drug is continued for two to three weeks or more. Thorazine also lowers the blood pressure, an effect which may manifest itself in a sensation of dizziness when a person stands up suddenly. In some people, Thorazine causes restlessness, a fixed facial expression, and trembling in the hands, arms or legs; these side effects, which resemble the symptoms of Parkinson's disease, can usually be controlled with an anti-Parkinsonian drug like Cogentin. A few people who have taken Thorazine for a long time experience an involuntary movement of the tongue and lips. Occasionally, thorazine can cause skin rash, jaundice, or a decrease in the white blood cell count which increases the patient's vulnerability to infection. The drug must then be discontinued.

precautions Prolonged use of Thorazine requires regular medical evaluation at intervals. There may be some interference with driving or operating machinery.

drug interactions Oversedation is possible when Thorazine is taken in combination with alcohol, other sedatives and tranquilizers, sleeping pills, antidepressants, antihistamines and drugs containing narcotics. If taken with the antihypertensive drugs Ismelin, and Aldomet, it can counteract their blood pressure-lowering effect. It can also cause constipation or bladder dysfunction in some if combined with antispasmodic drugs, anti-Parkinsonian drugs like Cogentin and tricyclic antidepressants like Elavil.

see essay *Major Tranquilizers.*

Thyroglobulin (generic name). See PROLOID.

Thyroid

trade names

Thyrolar, Thyrocrine

action and uses An extract from the thyroid glands of animals containing the natural thyroid hormones, sometimes called T-3 and

T-4. Thyroid hormones regulate many body functions, especially the metabolic rate (including the rate at which the cells of the body use oxygen). Thyroid is used to replace a hormone deficiency in diseases such as myxedema, and simple goiter. It has no place in weight control therapy. More recently, thyroid extract has been largely replaced by the pure hormones such as Synthroid.

adult dosage
There is no standard dose for thyroid. The dose must be individualized for each patient and depends on the results of tests of thyroid function and the response to the drug. The tablets come in 8 different strengths from 15 mg to 300 mg.

adverse effects
If too high a dose of thyroid is given, symptoms of overdose will occur. These include nervousness, sweating, irregular and rapid heartbeat, chest pains (angina) and, in women, irregular menstruation.

precautions
The required dose of thyroid may vary so regular checks of thyroid function may be needed. Careful regulation of the dose is important if high blood pressure or heart disease is also present.

drug interactions
When taken with thyroid drugs, certain tricyclic antidepressant drugs such as Elavil and decongestants or drugs for asthma can increase the likelihood of palpitations, rapid heart rate and elevation of the blood pressure.

see essay
Drugs for Thyroid Disorders.

Thyroxine (generic name). See SYNTHROID.

Tigan

generic name

trimethobenzamide hydrochloride

action and uses
A drug used for the control of nausea and vomiting. Tigan is often prescribed for the treatment of motion sickness and nausea and vomiting in other disorders. It should be used only when the cause of nausea is known. The exact way in which Tigan helps to control these symptoms is not known, but it is thought to act on the brain centre controlling vomiting.

adult dosage
Usually 250 mg three of four times per day, as needed. Tigan is also available as suppositories. The usual dose of these is one 200 mg suppository three or four times per day.

adverse effects
Side effects are relatively infrequent. Occasionally, however, drowsiness, skin rash, tremors of the hands, dizziness and headache may occur.

drug interactions | Tigan may be additive in its sedative effects to major or minor tranquilizers, sleeping pills or antihistamines.

see essay | *Drugs for Nausea, Stomach Upset and Ulcers.*

Tofranil

generic name

> imipramine (available by generic name)

action and uses | A commonly prescribed antidepressant drug. Like Elavil and Sinequan, Tofranil belongs to a group of closely-related drugs called tricyclic antidepressants, and is used to treat certain types of moderately severe and long-standing depression. The tricyclic antidepressants are not true tranquilizers, although they can cause some sedation. Though effective, the antidepressant effect of Tofranil may take days to weeks to appear, and a truly depressed person should be aware of this, as well as the initial side effects. Tofranil is sometimes used to treat childhood bedwetting.

adult dosage | The effective dose of Tofranil is highly individualized and dosage adjustment may take one or two months. Initially the dose is 50-100 mg per day, and may be increased to 150 or 200 mg per day. (The dose may be lower for elderly patients.) Because the drug is long-acting and may cause some sedation, it is usually taken just once a day, at bedtime.

adverse effects | Initially, Tofranil may cause dry mouth, blurred vision, drowsiness, constipation and difficulty in urination. These effects are especially a problem in older people, but they tend to disappear in 3-4 weeks. Other significant side effects may include effects on the heart rhythm, and sometimes confusion or dizziness.

precautions | Tofranil should be taken with caution by persons with glaucoma, prostate gland problems, liver or heart disease, epilepsy or hyperthyroid conditions. It should not be taken by pregnant or potentially pregnant or nursing women. The drowsiness may interfere with driving or operating machinery.

drug interactions | Tofranil can cause oversedation when taken in combination with alcohol, sleeping pills, tranquilizers, antihistamines and drugs containing narcotics. It can add to the side effects of drugs to lower blood pressure such as Ismelin. It can dangerously interfere with drugs to regulate heart rhythm, thyroid drugs and drugs of the MAO inhibitor family (such as Marplan, Parnate and Nardil). Taken with drugs of the latter type, or with the sedative

Placidyl, Tofranil can cause delirium.

Antidepressants.

see essay

Tolbutamide (generic name). See ORINASE.

Tolinase

generic name

tolazamide

action and uses
A drug which lowers glucose levels in the blood, used to treat diabetes. Because Tolinase can be taken orally (unlike insulin) it is termed an "oral hypoglycemic" drug. It is similar to other oral antidiabetic drugs such as Orinase and Diabinase, but not DBI. Tolinase works by stimulating the pancreas to produce insulin and by helping the cells to use glucose. It is only of value in diabetics who are able to make insulin. Such patients usually have mild diabetes which often becomes evident toward middle age (and is therefore known as maturity onset diabetes). Oral hypoglycemic drugs should only be taken if dietary measures alone have failed to control the condition. Resistance to the effects of Tolinase often develops after a few months to years. It is recommended that withdrawal of oral antidiabetic drugs be tried every six months to one year since their continued use may not be needed. The long term benefits versus risks of this and related drugs are now widely debated.

adult dosage
Dosage is individualized. Initially it is 100-250 mg daily with breakfast and adjustment is made according to response.

adverse effects
The most common and hazardous adverse effect is excessive *lowering* of the blood sugar, which can cause symptoms of dizziness, weakness, cold sweats and mental dullness. Older persons and those on several other drugs (see drug interactions below) or with liver or kidney disease are more prone to this. In proper dosage, other side effects are unusual, but rashes, blood or liver abnormalities and water retention can occur.

precautions
This drug should be avoided by pregnant or potentially pregnant and nursing women, as well as those with significant kidney, or liver disease. Those allergic to sulfa drugs may develop an allergy to this drug.

drug interactions
Thiazide diuretics (as hydrochlorothiazide, Diuril, Hygroton) can aggravate diabetes and may increase the dose requirement of the oral antidiabetic drug. A number of drugs can increase the risk of low blood sugar due to

increased levels of drug. These include insulin, sulfa drugs, anti-inflammatory drugs such as aspirin, Butazolidin and Tandearil and the anticonvulsant Dilantin. Inderal (propranolol) can also cause dangerous interactions and disguise the symptoms of hypoglycemia. Alcohol can cause a flushing reaction when taken with this drug.

see essay   *Drugs for Diabetes.*

Tranxene

generic name

> clorazepate

action and uses   A minor tranquilizer chemically related to Valium and Librium. Primarily used to relieve anxiety and nervous tension, Tranxene is also sometimes used to induce sleep and to treat the symptoms of alcohol withdrawal.

adult dosage   Usually 3.75 mg to 7.5 mg, 1 to 3 times per day. Because it is eliminated from the body rather slowly, it can also be taken once a day, at bedtime, in order to take advantage of its sleep-inducing effects. Accordingly, it is available in a once-daily dosage form, Tranxene SD which contains 22.5 mg (in other words, three 7.5 doses).

adverse effects   Drowsiness, dizziness and blurred vision are possible side effects with Tranxene, but these effects are usually dose-related, and can be reduced by lowering the dose. Though other side effects are possible, they are relatively unusual.

precautions   Because of the possible connection between similar drugs and birth defects, Tranxene should not be used by pregnant or potentially pregnant women.

drug dependence   It may interfere with driving or operating machinery. Prolonged use of Tranxene may cause habituation and withdrawal symptoms when discontinued.

drug interactions   The sedative effects of Tranxene can be increased by alcohol, antihistamines, sleeping pills, and other sedatives, tranquilizers and antidepressants.

see essay   *Minor Tranquilizers.*

Triamcinolone (generic name). See ARISTOCORT, KENALOG.

Triavil

generic ingredients

> antidepressant = amitriptyline
> major tranquilizer = perphenazine

action and uses   A combination drug promoted and used to treat moderate to severe anxiety with depression. Triavil contains two potent drugs: amitriptyline, a tricyclic antidepressant used in the treatment of moderate to severe depression; and perphenazine, an antipsychotic drug, or major tranquilizer, used in the treatment of psychoses, or thought disorders. There is some question among medical authorities as to the rationale behind the use of these two drugs in a fixed combination form.

In the first place, when used alone, both drugs require careful individualized dosage adjustment, something which cannot be done with any subtlety when they are combined. (Raising or lowering the dose of one drug in a fixed combination automatically alters the dose of the other as well.) Secondly, the adverse effects of the two drugs (described below) are very similar and can be additive. Thirdly, although Triavil is promoted for the treatment of anxiety with depression, neither of its two components is a true anti-anxiety drug. One rationale for the use of this combination drug is that the antidepressant amitriptyline will on occasion produce a thought disorder which can be suppressed by perphenazine, but whether this is true has not been carefully established in clinical testing. In the final analysis, it is questionable whether, in view of their additive side effects, the use of these two potent drugs is justified in any but truly serious mental disorders, and then it is possible that only one is truly indicated.

adult dosage   Triavil is available in four tablet sizes, which are recommended 3-4 times per day, but since both ingredients are long-acting, they can be taken once daily, usually in the evening to use the sedative effect.

adverse effects   Triavil has the combined side effects of its two components, which in this case are significant and additive. Amitriptyline and perphenazine can both cause dry mouth, blurred vision, urine retention, constipation and rapid or irregular heartbeat. Perphenazine can also cause Parkinsonian symptoms (a rigid facial expression, stiff gait, and trembling in the hands, arms and feet), as well as dizziness, jaundice, blood disorders and severe skin rashes.

precautions   Triavil should not be used by pregnant, potentially pregnant or nursing women. Triavil should be used with caution by patients with glaucoma, prostate gland trouble, heart disease, epilepsy, impaired liver function, or hyperthyroidism.

drug interactions   Oversedation is possible when Triavil is combined with alcohol, other tranquilizers and antidepressants, sleeping pills, sedatives, and drugs containing narcotics. The amitriptyline in Triavil can interfere with drugs to lower blood pressure, thyroid drugs of the MAO inhibitor family (such as Marplan, Parnate and Nardil). The perphenazine in Triavil can also dangerously interfere with drugs to lower blood pressure. Both drugs can be additive to antispasmodic drugs and anti-Parkinsonian drugs such as Cogentin to cause constipation.

see essay *Major Tranquilizers and Antidepressants.*

Trihexyphenidyl (generic name). See ARTANE.

Tri-Vi-Flor

generic ingredients

vitamins = A, D, C
mineral = fluoride

action and uses A fixed combination vitamin-mineral supplement used for infants. The vitamins are used to supplement the regular food of infants. The flouride is used to help prevent dental cavities, when there is no flouride in the water supply.

dosage Usually 1 dropperful (1 ml per day) of the drops or 1 tablet daily of the chewable tablets.

adverse effects Both vitamins A and D can cause serious adverse effects if taken in excess. Vitamin A can cause liver and skin abnormalities, vitamin D, bone abnormalities.

precautions Tri-Vi-Flor should not be used if the local community water already contains fluoride. Only the dose recommended should be used, preferably with a doctor's advice.

drug interactions No significant interactions occur at the recommended dose.

see essay *Vitamins and Minerals.*

Tuss-Ornade

generic ingredients

cough suppressant
and anticholinergic = caramiphen
antihistamine = chlorpheniramine
decongestant = phenylpropanolamine
anticholinergic = isopropamide iodide

action and uses This mixture of ingredients is available as a long-acting, time-released Spansule or as a liquid; it is identical to Ornade, except for the addition of ingredients which can decrease coughing and have a drying (anticholinergic) action. Its effect on decreasing cough is less than that of codeine, but because there is some cough suppressant effect, Tuss-Ornade should be primarily reserved for occasions when that effect is desired. The other ingredients are directed to relieving symptoms of nasal stuffiness and a runny nose.

adult dosage
Spansule: One capsule every 12 hours hours as needed for symptoms. Liquid: 1-2 teaspoons 3-4 times per day.

adverse effects
Drowsiness may occur due to the antihistamine and the caramiphen, and the anticholingergic drugs may cause an excessively dry nose and mouth. There may be palpitations or dizziness. Persons with heart disease or high blood pressure, diabetes or prostate trouble may be more susceptible to these effects.

precautions
This drug should be avoided by pregnant, potentially pregnant and nursing women. This drug should not be taken by a person allergic to iodine. Because the preparation may decrease alertness, driving or operating machinery may be hazardous. Those with heart trouble or high blood pressure should check with their doctor since this drug can increase blood pressure.

drug interactions
Both the antihistaminic and the antitussive (cough suppressant) sedative effects can add to the effects of alcohol and tranquilizing drugs. The anticholinergic effects (dry mouth or bladder problems) of the two components can be additive to antispasmodic drugs (such as Pro-Banthine or Librax) and tricyclic antidepressant drugs such as Elavil. The iodide present can interfere with tests of thyroid function.

see essay
Drugs for Cough and Colds.

Tylenol

generic name
| acetaminophen (available by generic name) |

Tylenol with Codeine

generic ingredients
| narcotic = codeine
pain reliever = acetaminophen |

action and uses
A popular, mild analgesic drug avialable with and without the addition of codeine, a narcotic analgesic. With codeine it is used to treat more severe pain than can be relieved by simple analgesics such as aspirin or acetaminophen.

adult dosage
One or two tablets, every 4-6 hours as needed for pain.

adverse effects
The major side effects which can occur are due to the

codeine, which can cause constipation, occasional nausea and vomiting, and occasionally dizziness. Large doses of acetaminophen can cause serious liver disease.

precautions

Because habitual use is a hazard, the forms containing codeine should be used only when non-narcotic analgesics are not effective.

drug dependence

Prolonged use of codeine may cause dependence.

drug interactions

The codeine effect can be additive to other narcotic drugs as well as to other sedating drugs such as tranquilizers or alcohol.

see essay

Narcotic Pain Relievers.

Valisone cream, ointment, lotion and spray

generic name

betamethasone

action and uses

A commomly used topical preparation of a synthetic corticosteroid, or cortisone-like drug. It is used primarliy because of its anti-inflammatory effects in the treatment of many types of skin disorders such as psoriasis, certain types of neurodermatitis and a variety of other conditions where there is no infection. In many cases, the effects are dramatic. Because it retards formation of scar tissue, it can also prevent scarring.

adult dosage

The preparation is applied sparingly 2-3 times daily. It is available in ointments, lotions, creams and a spray, in several strengths, depending upon where it is to be used.

adverse effects

If the preparation is not used for long periods or on infected areas, there are virtually no important adverse effects; however, if the preparations are used for long intervals on the face, they can cause eruptions and redness. If Valisone preparations are used for long periods on a large portion of the body, the corticosteroid can be absorbed and get into the body. This can cause weight gain, ulcers or stomach upset, decreased resistance to infection and stress, and can be quite hazardous. If used on an infected area of the skin it can help the infection spread, and it can be very hazardous if used for any viral skin lesions such as herpes (cold sores), shingles or chickenpox.

precautions

Do not use for long periods of time or on large areas of the body except under continued medical supervision. If a skin eruption worsens with continued use, the physician should be notified and the preparation discontinued.

drug interactions

No significant interactions will occur although other

topical preparations placed on the same skin area may interfere with effects.

see essays

Steroids or Cortisone-like Drugs. Drugs for Skin and Local Disorders.

Valium

generic name

> diazepam

action and uses

A minor tranquilizer widely used to treat anxiety and nervousness. The primary effect of Valium is to produce calm and decrease the feeling of anxiety. Valium together with related drugs such as Librium, Serax, Dalmane and Tranxene, is one of a group of drugs which are the most frequently prescribed in the United States. Valium is usually prescribed to relieve the symptoms of a condition in the same way that narcotics are used to relieve pain. In general it has no effect on the cause of the symptoms. Valium is also often used in the treatment of withdrawal from certain drugs, especially alcohol. It can also be used as a sleeping medication in a similar way to the related drug, Dalmane. It is not known exactly how these drugs work.

adult dosage

The usual dose of Valium ranges from 10 mg per day to 2-10 mg, 2 to 4 times per day, depending on individual requirements. Some people are strongly sedated by 2-5 mg, while others are not especially effected by that dose.

adverse effects

The most common side effect of Valium is sedation and depression, and sometimes, dizziness, but this can usually be relieved by lowering the dosage. Other side effects are relatively uncommon. A few individuals may suffer from increased anxiety when taking Valium, but this is rare. When Valium is taken in combination with alcohol the two drugs act together and marked sedation may occur.

drug dependence

Valium is not additive in the same way as narcotics but, like other sedatives, it can be habit-forming to a certain extent if taken for a long period of time. If it is then stopped suddenly some withdrawal symptoms may occur, especially after large doses. These can include anxiety, insomnia and nightmares. In some cases the sedation may interfere with working and driving.

precautions

There is a possibility that minor tranquilizers may cause birth defects and the manufacturers therefore warn against the use of Valium in pregnant or potentially pregnant women.

drug interactions   Valium can enhance the sedative effect of alcohol, antihistamines, sleeping pills and narcotics, sometimes to a dangerous extent. Unlike many sedatives, Valium does not interfere with the actions of the anticoagulant, Coumadin.

see essay   *Minor Tranquilizers.*

Vasodilan

generic name

> isoxsuprine (available by generic name)

action and uses   This drug is promoted and used for disorders causing decreased circulation to the brain, feet or hands. Although it relaxes normal blood vessels (and therefore increases the flow of blood) in the muscles of the extremities, there is no clear evidence that in can increase blood flow in abnormal states, such as when there is arteriosclerosis (fatty obstruction) of the blood vessels, or when a person experiences coldness of the extremities or pain with exercise (intermittent claudication). It is also used, but is questionably effective, in conditions where there is temporary spasm of the arteries, such as Raynaud's phenomenon.

adult dosage   10-20 mg 3 to 4 times a day.

adverse effects   Vasodilan is well tolerated, but may cause dizziness, especially with rapid change in position, and rapid heart rate. Allergic rashes may also occur.

precautions   This drug should not be used directly after minor or major surgery or childbirth. It should be avoided by pregnant or potentially pregnant women.

drug interactions   Vasodilan may add to effects of other more effective blood-vessel relaxing drugs, such as nitroglycerin or Apresoline, to lower blood pressure.

see essay   *Drugs used to Prevent or Treat Circulation Disorders.*

V-Cillin K

generic name

> phenoxymethyl penicillin (available by generic name)

action and uses   A semi-synthetic penicillin antibiotic which is almost identical to penicillin G in its action and adverse effects except that due to a small difference in its chemical structure, it is more effective orally. This is because it is not easily destroyed by stomach acid. V-Cillin K acts to prevent formation of the cell walls of bacteria. This prevents their growth and multiplication. There is no effect on human cells due to differences in structure. It is most

effective against the group of bacteria which commonly cause sore throats ("strep" throat), pneumonia and certain abcesses, although some bacteria in abcesses (staphylococci or "staph") can become resistant to penicillin G, especially in hospitals. V-Cillin K, like the other penicillins, is not as effective for treatment of serious infections by the group of bacteria called Gram negative bacilli, which cause infections in the urinary tract, bowel and elsewhere. It has no effect on virus or fungal infections.

adult dosage
The usual oral dose is 250-500 mg (equivalent to 0.4-0.8 million units) every six hours on an empty stomach, but this is individualized, according to the infection.

adverse effects
The most common adverse effect is gastrointestinal upset, cramps or diarrhea. Given by injection or orally, the primary concern is the occurrence of allergic reactions, which can include skin rashes or hives, swelling of the face or throat, difficulty breathing, or some time later, joint pains and fever.

precautions
V-Cillin K should not be taken when there is known allergy to any of the penicillin drugs. Once a course of V-Cillin K is prescribed, it should be taken for the prescribed length of time (usually 5-10 days) even though symptoms may disappear. This is very important since the infection may otherwise recur and even develop resistance to the antibiotic.

drug interactions
In some cases, the effect of V-Cillin K may be decreased if erythromycin or chloramphenicol is also taken.

see essay
Drugs to Treat Infections.

Vibramycin

generic name

doxycycline (available by generic name)

action and uses
A slightly different and more costly form of one of the most commonly used oral antibiotics, tetracycline. There are a number of tetracycline drugs available, but most are comparable in their actions and side effects except for Vibramycin and Minocin. Doxycycline is known as a "broad spectrum" antibiotic because it can be used in a wide variety of different infections, although it is the first choice drug in very few common infections. It acts by stopping the production of proteins in sensitive bacterial cells with little effect on human cells. Doxycycline

sometimes is used by those with chronic bronchitis or other lung disease, for other minor infections and occasionally for acne. Because of its cost, it often is reserved for use as an alternate to tetracycline when kidney disease is present since it does not harm the diseased kidney like other tetracyclines.

adult dosage

The dose and schedule for doxycycline is also different from other tetracyclines. The usual oral dose is 100-200 mg the first day, then 50-100 mg once or twice a day for a prescribed number of days as specified by the physician. It is very important to take this on an empty stomach. The dose may vary in some cases such as acne, where it may be lower.

adverse effects

Doxycycline can cause various gastrointestinal symptoms including nausea and vomiting, burning stomach or belching, cramps and diarrhea. The latter symptom, due to the fact that tetracycline inhibits some bacteria in the lower intestine and elsewhere and allows overgrowth of other bacteria and minor fungi, may be less frequent with doxycycline. These symptoms tend to disappear when the drug is discontinued. Less commonly, tetracycline can cause rashes. or other allergic reactions and sensitivity of the skin to sunlight, causing rashes (photosensitivity). It can also rarely cause liver damage or blood cell abnormalities.

precautions

Doxycycline should not be taken by pregnant or potentially preganant or nursing women, and should be used with caution when significant liver disease is present. This antibiotic, like all others, should be taken for the time period directed, and every dose should be taken. Failure to do this can result in inadequate treatment of the infection, recurrence or development of resistant infections.

drug interactions

The most common drug interaction is between the tetracycline and antacids or milk products, since the tetracycline can bind to these and does not get into the body. Doxycycline can potentially increase the effect of the anticoagulant Coumadin and increase the hazard of bleeding.

see essay

Drugs to Treat Infections.

Vioform-Hydrocortisone

generic ingredients

antibacterial/antifungal = iodochlorohydroxyquin corticosteroid = hydrocortisone

action and uses

A topical preparation used to treat a wide variety of skin

conditions associated with local infection of the skin, including various types of eczema, and fungal infections of the foot (athlete's foot) and of other areas. The preparation is available without the steroid as Vioform. There is some controversy whether addition of the hydrocortisone (which as a corticosteroid, does decrease inflammation and scarring) is useful or not, since it may help spread the infection. It is available as a cream, lotion or ointment, depending on where it is to be used. Ointments are customarily used on dry areas, lotions on moist areas.

adult dosage The preparation of 3% iodochlorhydroxyquin and 1% hydrocortisone is applied sparingly to the affected area 3-4 times daily.

adverse effects Allergies can occur to the ointment which may be hard to detect, except when there is failure of an area to heal and increased itching. Both ingredients may be absorbed into the body if used on large areas for long periods. This can cause interference with tests of thyroid function due to the iodine-containing product. Long-term absorption of the hydrocortisone can also cause weight gain, stomach upset or ulcer, and decreased resistance to infection or illness. Very long-term use can also cause local breakdown of the skin (similar to stretch marks).

precautions Do not use for long periods of time or on large areas of the body except under continued medical supervision. If a skin eruption worsens with continued use, the physician should be notified and the preparation discontinued.

drug interactions The iodine-containing compound can interfere with tests of thyroid.

see essays *Steroids or Cortisone-like Drugs. Drugs for Skin and Local Disorders.*

Vistaril

generic name

> hydroxyzine

action and uses An antihistamine which is primarily promoted for its anti-anxiety and sedating actions. It has a chemical structure similar to other antihistamines such as Marezine, which are used for motion sickness, and it is essentially identical to the drug Atarax. Vistaril is also used on occasion as an antihistamine and in the treatment of conditions which cause itching of the skin.

adult dosage Because sensitivity to its effect varies, the dose ranges from 25 to 100 mg 2 to 3 times a day.

adverse effects Excessive sedation or decreased mental alertness may create a significant problem. Other side effects are relatively unusual.

precuations
Vistaril may interfere with driving or operating machinery. It should not be used by pregnant, potentially pregnant or nursing women.

drug interactions
Vistaril is additive to other drugs causing sedation, such as sleeping pills, tranquilizers, alcohol and narcotics such as morphine; these combinations should be avoided unless a greater degree of sedation is desired.

see essays
Antihistamines. Minor Tranquilizers.

Zyloprim

generic name
allopurinol

action and uses
A drug used in the treatment of gout. Zyloprim is a chemical which helps to lower the level of uric acid in the blood. If uric acid levels rise too high, crystals of uric acid salts collect in joints and other places, especially the big toes and ears, to form deposits called tophi. It can also gradually destroy the joints, and also form crystals in the kidneys to cause stones. This general condition is known as gout. Zyloprim prevents uric acid from forming and thus prevents the deposition of the crystals in the joints, and in the kidneys. It is also used to reduce uric acid levels in other diseases such as leukemia, cancer and kidney disease.

adult dosage
The average dose is 200 to 300 mg per day, in a single dose, with adjustment made according to uric acid levels in the blood.

adverse effects
Some people develop sensitivity to Zyloprim and may suffer from skin rash, itching or hives. Severe allergic reactions can develop. Drowsiness, and liver abnormalities may also occur. When the drug is first started, acute attacks of gout may be produced, so another antigout drug, colchicine, is usually added for several days to prevent this.

precautions
Zyloprim should not be used during pregnancy or by nursing mothers. The dosage must be adjusted when taken with certain other drugs used for tumors or to suppress immunity.

drug interactions
Zyloprim can increase the effect of the anti coagulants Coumadin,Dicumarol and some other drugs. The dose of Zyloprim may need to be decreased when the drugs mercaptopurine and Immuran are also used.

see essay
Drugs for Gout.